The GOLFER'S GUIDE
to **PILATES**

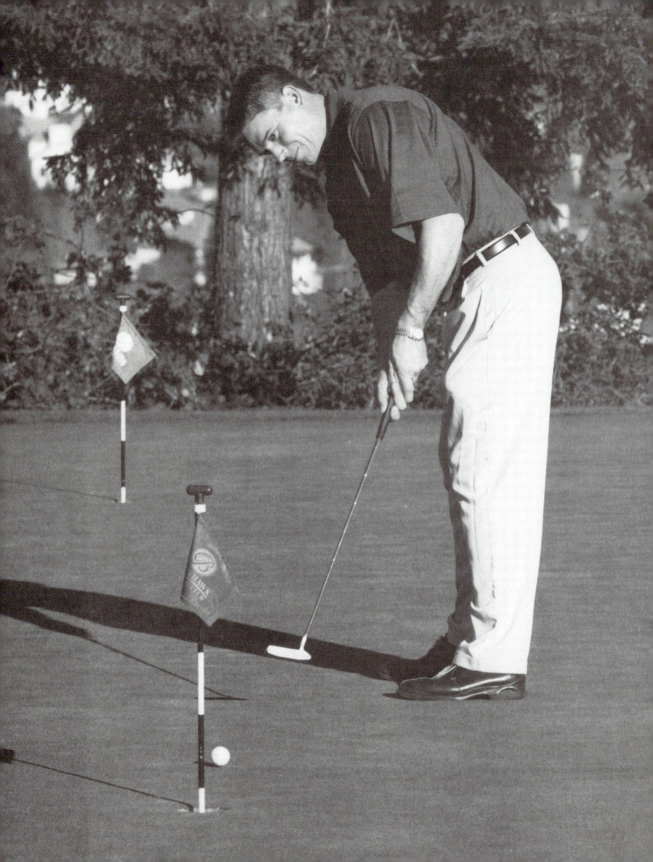

The GOLFER'S GUIDE
to PILATES

**Step-by-Step Exercises
to Strengthen Your Game**

Monica Clyde

photography by Robert Holmes

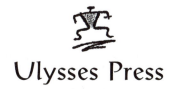

Ulysses Press

Published in the United States by Ulysses Press
P.O. Box 3440
Berkeley, CA 94703
www.ulyssespress.com

ISBN 1-56975-538-8
Library of Congress Control Number 2006900286

Printed in Canada by Webcom

10 9 8 7 6 5 4 3 2 1

Editorial/Production	Lily Chou, Claire Chun, Steven Zah Schwartz, Matt Orendorff
Index	Sayre Van Young
Cover design	DiAnna VanEycke
Interior photographs	Robert Holmes except on pages 11, 12, 14, 20, 23, 28, 30 & 119 © photos.com
Cover photographs	*front:* © photos.com (top) and Robert Holmes (bottom); *back:* Robert Holmes
Models	Monica Clyde, Dylan Hills, Louise McMenamin, Kerry Silverstone

Distributed by Publishers Group West

Please Note
This book has been written and published strictly for informational purposes, and in no way should be used as a substitute for consultation with health care professionals. You should not consider educational material herein to be the practice of medicine or to replace consultation with a physician or other medical practitioner. The author and publisher are providing you with information in this work so that you can have the knowledge and can choose, at your own risk, to act on that knowledge. The author and publisher also urge all readers to be aware of their health status and to consult health care professionals before beginning any health program.

To my husband Barry,
who brings out the best in me

contents

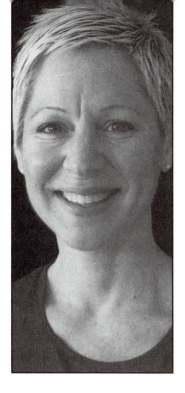

preface

I live on a golf course in a lovely community. We commonly see our neighbors as we gather in our backyards overlooking the golf course. One evening my neighbor Joan and I were chatting and watching our husbands swing with a new golf-training toy. "He says this is going to give him a whole new game," she said with a wry smile. "The Holy Grail of golf."

We laughed at the thought of us all buying into the idea that something "out there" will solve all of our golf imperfections.

I wrote this book because I believe this program can give golfers more of what they're looking for. I know *The Golfer's Guide to Pilates* program is not the Holy Grail of golf. However, the program put forth in this book can significantly enhance your golfing experience while extending your years of play. It's not quick or easy, and in fact takes patience, perseverance and commitment; it requires many of the same qualities as golf. But with consistency and practice you can develop the body-mind equip-

ment you already own and the qualities that will soon become evident in your life, your scores and in your enjoyment of the game.

I have a background as a dancer, body therapist, movement therapist, personal trainer, Master Pilates Instructor and a lifelong athlete. As an adult, I began experimenting with different movement forms. I was quite taken with a variety of martial arts forms because the training was not just for the body, but a way of linking or synchronizing the body and the mind for physical and mental performance.

I decided to learn to play golf in my early 40s, bringing my vast movement background

with me. I began by taking golf lessons that taught me about swing mechanics. However, I also indulged my passion for movement and delved into the study of golf movement biomechanics as well as the kinesiology and the mind-body requirements of the game. Instead of paying attention to where the club needed to be, I focused on where my body and mind needed to be to produce certain swing results. It's an internal rather than external focus. I call it "playing from the inside out."

I quickly understood the underlying challenges inherent in the movements required by golf. Most people are weak where they need to be strong and tight where they need to be flexible. What a set up for frustration and injury! I realized that golf lessons teach swing mechanics but don't address the issues of biomechanics other than to teach golfers how to compensate for their lack of biomechanical ability. It was evident immediately that the Pilates Method was a perfect training form for golfers because it trains the mind and body synergistically and functionally, just like martial

arts or dance training, for performance.

This program produces golfers who gain distance and accuracy, and who play without pain or discomfort. In addition, all of them enjoy their game and their golfing lifestyle more.

When you consider your mind and body as your best equipment, you'll learn to keep them well conditioned and tuned for your game. With a bit of time and a lot of commitment,

you can feel and play your best.

One of my clients, Steve, is a wonderful athlete and a scratch golfer. During a training session one day, he paused and said, "This training is doing great things for my game right now, but I was thinking, even more important is what it'll do for the longevity of my game. I'll be able to play golf with my family for a very long time, and that makes me happy."

And that is why I wrote this book.

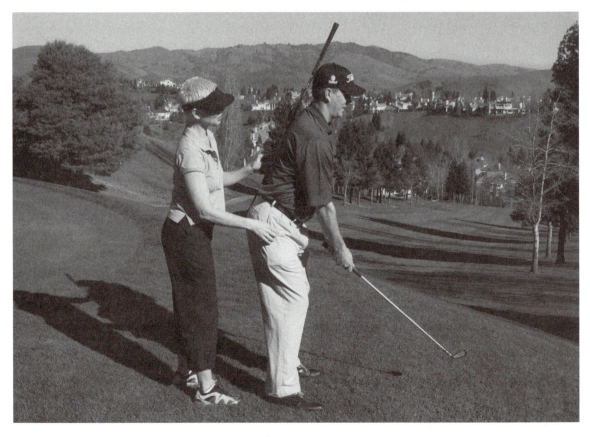

Author Monica Clyde helps Dylan find his proper spine angle.

part one:

getting started

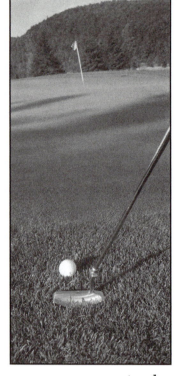

pilates for golf

Welcome to *The Golfer's Guide to Pilates*, the Pilates Method of conditioning for golf. Congratulations on taking the initiative to pursue a better game and a better body! As a golfer, you already possess the finest piece of golf equipment in the world: your body-mind.

When finely tuned and synchronized, your body-mind will do more to enhance your golf game than anything you can purchase. Golfers spend millions of dollars on equipment and lessons each year, yet continue to suffer from the same swing faults, playing challenges and injuries. This is because many swing faults and playing challenges are due to physical and mental imbalances, not faulty equipment.

Historically, most golfers play golf to get into shape to play golf. The importance of golf-specific conditioning is just now beginning to be widely accepted, partly due, in my opinion, to Tiger Woods. When Tiger appeared on the golf scene, we began to hear the words "golf" and "athlete" in the same sentence. With this new athletic approach to the sport, golfers are beginning to understand how physically and mentally demanding their sport is and are achieving significant improvements in performance through golf-specific training, both physical and mental.

Most professional athletes engage in some kind of formal conditioning that prepares the mind and body for their game. They understand the difference between conditioning for the sport and *playing* the sport. And many of the world's greatest athletes and performers use the Pilates Method as an integral part of their conditioning program because it gives students the mental and physical edge they need to be at the top of their game. Playing golf doesn't develop your body or your mind to its fullest potential for the game, but mind-body conditioning for golf does.

The Golfer's Guide to Pilates will optimize your physical and mental game with a step-by-step golf-specific instruction program that blends the most effective, cutting-edge training available. With this program, you'll learn the movement of golf and also develop the blend of flexibility and strength you need to play. You'll learn to move in a way that leads to consistency, accuracy and increased club-head speed for longer distance. Part of what makes this program so unique among training programs is that while you're conditioning your body and mind for golf, you're also developing a very healthy physique and a heightened sense of well-being.

Building better bodies and minds is the original purpose of the Pilates Method. When your body and mind are well conditioned, the risk of injury is reduced while the longevity of your play is increased. Make the most of the equipment you already possess, your body and your mind. You'll move, play and feel better when your game

is complete. This book will show you how to develop your mind and body for the life of your game and the game of your life.

About the Pilates Method

Joseph H. Pilates developed the Pilates Method in the early 1900s and opened the first Pilates studio in the United States in New York City in 1926. Though frail and sickly as a child due to asthma and other complications, through his "zest for life" and a determination to build a strong physique, he studied and practiced different movement forms. Joe understood that the body moves as an integrated whole rather than in isolated parts, and was aware of the mind-body connection well before it became cliché. "It is the mind

itself that controls the body" is one of his most famous sayings.

Joe developed a movement methodology originally named Contrology, in which the principles of concentration, control, breath, center, precision, fluidity, imagery and intuition became the basis for practicing what became known as the Pilates Method exercises. His series of mat exercises was designed to build balance and symmetry, which are paramount to a sense of well-being and true strength. The Pilates mat exercises use one's own body weight to simultaneously develop flexibility and strength, especially in the abdominals, back, buttocks and the smaller, deeper muscles that give support to the bones and joints. Nowadays, those muscles are called the "core." Joe under-

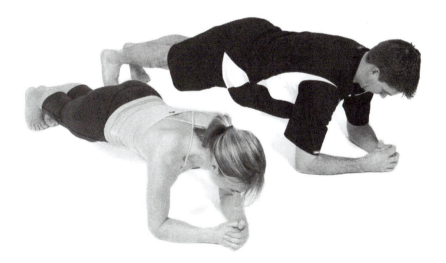

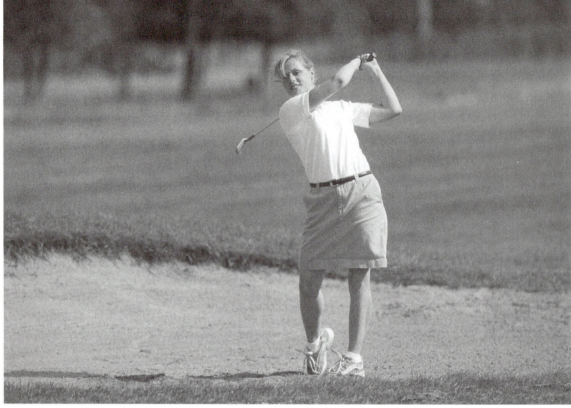

stood that the core muscles are those from which true integrity and strength stem. He even named the muscles of the lower abdominal region "the power-house," indicating that all true power comes from the core.

The Pilates exercises and repertoire continue to evolve as the science of movement and motor-skill development advance. Today there are a number of training institutions based upon the Pilates Method. Some are classical and focus strictly on the original Pilates exercises and formats; others have evolved to include more functional uses for the Pilates exercises, such as standing work and the use of small apparatus tools like the foam roller and the elastic exercise band.

Pilates continues to be one of the fastest-growing segments of the fitness and rehabilitation industry. Each year more and more physical therapists attend my trainings to learn the specifics of working with golfers. They understand the value of Pilates-based exercises, especially for their golfer clientele. While the Pilates Method is enjoying rapid growth these days, it is not a fad. Rather, Joe was way ahead of his time and we're just catching up. The reason the Pilates Method has become so popular is really very simple—it works! Moreover, it just so happens that it's particularly suited to the needs of golfers, which is why some of the world's greatest golfers, like Tiger and Annika, use the Pilates Method as an integral part of their golf training program.

The more often you practice the Pilates Method, the more quickly the principles will become integrated into your day-to-day life and movements. After a month or two of regular training, the concepts and principles will integrate and align your body and mind. At this point, your fellow golfers will begin to ask you what you are doing to improve your game.

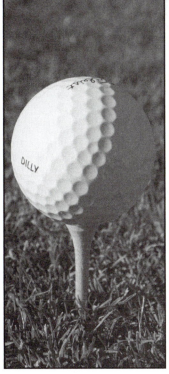

body-mind training

Golf is a body-mind sport. We analyze each shot for a series of variables, including the lie of the ball, the distance to the hole, obstacles and air quality. Then we visualize the best way to advance the ball toward and into the hole. The image of the shot is then relayed from the mind to body in order to shape a swing or stroke to carry out the intended shot we imagined. The best results come when the mind and body are synchronized, working together to carry out the actions you imagined for your shot.

It sounds so easy, but we all know the results are not always what we had imagined. What makes golf so challenging is that it requires us to stay focused mentally and to move precisely, and then repeat that focused precision consistently. Golfers need a new paradigm for training, one that builds precision and fluidity with power and focus rather than just strong muscles.

Watch gymnasts on the horse or on the rings—they move with power, fluidity and precision, and

have incredible focus and intent. Another great example of power and precision can be found in martial arts training. You've probably seen martial artists on television or perhaps even in person. They can jump, spin, kick and land, knowing exactly where they are in space *and* be prepared for the next series of movements. This requires speed, power and precision.

To learn to move with speed, power, agility and precision, a golfer needs to begin training

with small, repetitive movements, just like a martial artist. At the same time, he/she begins training the mind in the art of concentration and mindfulness in movement, as well as learning how to use his/her physical and mental energy. It's the blending of mind and body in movement. I call it the "wax on/wax off" principle, which comes from the 1980s movie, *The Karate Kid.*

In the film, a young man named Daniel wanted to learn

karate to protect himself from neighborhood bullies. Mr. Miyagi, the handyman at Daniel's apartment complex, just happened to be a karate master and agreed to train him. Daniel's grand ideas about learning fancy kicks and punches were quickly dashed, however, when Mr. Miyagi first had the boy perform menial tasks around his home. Daniel spent his entire first day of "training" waxing Mr. Miyagi's collection of old, dusty cars. Mr. Miyagi was very particular about how Daniel should go about doing this waxing job, circling one arm one way to put the wax on, and circling the other arm the opposite way to take the wax off. Thus "wax on/wax off."

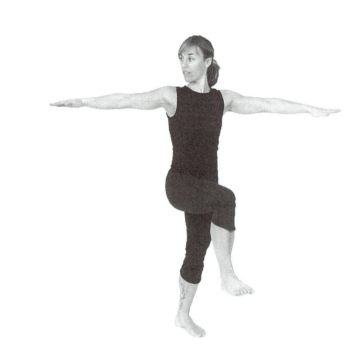

That evening, when Daniel finished waxing the cars, he expected some karate training. To his dismay, Mr. Miyagi only praised his work and told him to return tomorrow. Over the course of the next two days, Daniel painted the fence, then sanded the deck by hand. Finally, with his arms sore from three days of manual labor, Daniel angrily confronted Mr. Miyagi. "I am here to learn karate, not to do your chores!"

Only then did Mr. Miyagi reveal to Daniel that he had already learned some of the essential mental and physical requirements of karate. He had overcome the mental hazards of frustration and hurry and had developed focus, patience and perseverance. Moreover, he had begun to develop his physique for karate because all of the hand and arm movements he had learned while waxing, painting and sanding translated into the basic karate movements for defending himself. The moral of the "wax on/wax off" story for golfers: The small steps that seemingly have nothing to do with your goal will get you there faster than anything else will.

Legendary golfer Ben Hogan described the same process as learning to play the piano. You begin by playing scales repeat-edly to develop movement skills, tempo, rhythm and fluid-ity. It may seem simplistic but eventually, by putting the notes together in different sequences, you make music.

This "wax on/wax off" approach makes the program in *The Golfer's Guide to Pilates* unique. It takes a little longer and requires commitment, but the results will speak for them-selves. In the Pilates world, we have a saying: "In 10 sessions you will feel the difference, in 20 sessions you will see the difference and in 30 sessions you will have a new body." The same is true for golfers, except that you can add, "In 30 sessions you will have a new body *and* a new game."

Fully
Functional Training

If you have golfed for any length of time, you've probably experienced those elusive, "perfect shot" moments—when everything seemingly comes together, when your mind is clear of chatter and your swing is free and effortless. In those moments, our body and mind are synchronized and our swing movements, our tempo, and the firing sequence of all of our muscles are integrated, efficient and powerful. Those are the moments that keep us coming back for more.

Integrated movement is the focus of functionally based training. Traditional body-building techniques had a very different focus than the current methods used by athletes today, yet many people are still training with the body-building paradigm. Body-building techniques were originally developed with the purpose of increasing muscle mass for contests. The muscles are worked in a way that causes them to grow in bulk. This kind of workout stresses muscle isolation, working one muscle or muscle group individually to the point of fatigue. The weight workouts and workout machines found at many gyms still reflect the body-building

paradigm, but a new fitness paradigm called functional training, based upon the scientific study of motor-skill development, is beginning to take its place.

The body does not move in isolation; rather, the muscles, joints and nervous system all work in harmony to generate efficient and powerful movement. Functional training is based upon the way the nervous system works in connection with other systems to maintain center of gravity and create efficient movement patterns. The functional model has been used in the physical therapy world and is finally making its way into the fitness world.

Golfers need to understand the difference between the types of training because in order to have an efficient and powerful swing, all systems need to be trained. The Pilates repertoire simultaneously builds balance, strength and flexibility, while teaching the body to move in integrated, efficient ways. If you watch some of the better golfers

swing, you'll see power, but if you look even more closely, you'll see that they possess a certain grace that only comes from holistic, integrated movement patterns.

This program combines classical Pilates principles and exercises with functional-training principles and movements. Most golfers see and feel a difference in their body and their game soon after embarking on this Pilates-based program. It is not, however, a quick fix. To play and feel your best, you must be willing to commit to a consistent training regimen. The mind and the body blend and synchronize with time and constant attention. Think of your workouts like going to the practice range. Regular visits to the practice range give you the opportunity to focus on perfecting your swing mechanics. A regular workout gives you the opportunity to perfect your golf biomechanics and also increase power, agility and finesse.

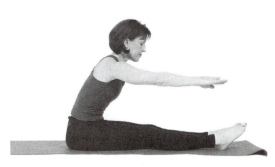

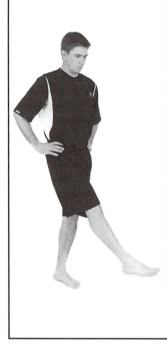

the principles of power

The power of Pilates lies within its principles of intelligent movement. These principles, when practiced consistently and with deep intention during your movement exercise sessions, synchronize mind and body.

Breath

Attention to the breath is first and foremost in all exercises and movement. Noticing your breath brings your awareness to your body and synchronizes mind and body to work together. Your breath is also a source of core strength and power. Think of the martial artist who exhales audibly when executing a powerful movement. Many tennis players also use the audible exhale to draw a bit more power out of their body and into their swing.

The breath is one of the most effective ways to enhance your game. Because breathing is something we do everyday, all day long, we have a tendency to take it for granted. People commonly hold their breath without even realizing it. If you've never engaged in any kind of formal breathing exercises, you may not have experienced the energy and power that comes from proper breathing.

It's a principle of movement that fluid movement requires a fluid breathing pattern. Proper breathing also assists in regulating oxygen levels in the brain and tissues, enhancing mental acuity, releasing tension in the body and maintaining a calm yet energized system.

Golfers can draw upon the awesome power of the breath by inhaling on the backswing and exhaling on the downswing and follow-through. For putting, inhale on the way back and exhale on the way through. The forced exhale activates the abdominal muscles, which in turn increases the amount of core power within the swing. When used in this fashion, you can use your breath to access physical power and energy.

The Pilates breath also stretches the small muscles in between the ribs, called intercostals. This is great for golfers because the area of the torso where the ribs are has the least amount of flexibility in the entire spine. Stretching the intercostal muscles increases a golfer's ability to rotate. As the ribcage gains flexibility and movement, the ability to rotate is enhanced. Increased breath control along with greater rotation equals more power in your swing.

The Pilates breath is designed to oxygenate your system, create power and fluidity in your movement, and keep you energized. If you suffer from asthma or other respiratory problems, you may require additional time to get accustomed to the Pilates breath. Asthmatics often do what is called "accessory breathing," which means using extra muscles (accessory muscles) to attempt to increase lung expansion. You'll greatly benefit from the Pilates breath by learning to release some of the extraneous muscle energy and gain control of your breathing pattern and therefore your swing pattern. The Pilates breathing technique will be covered in depth in Part 3 (see pages 58–60).

Concentration

Concentration means absolute focus and deep intention on each and every movement—focus the mind on the body and it will respond. Concentration builds mental stamina, keeping you from becoming caught up in distractions or from mentally "falling apart." It's said that Tiger Woods has a tremendous mental game due to his ability to focus and concentrate, a skill he learned from his mother, a Buddhist. Practice the art of concentration regularly with your exercise program and you'll develop mental stamina for your game. When concentration is broken, come back to the breath, which will reestablish the mind-body connection and return your focus to the movement.

Control

Each movement is practiced with utmost control. There is no place for sloppy movement. Small, controlled movements grow into fuller and more powerful movements. The martial artist has trained for ultimate control and power. Ben Hogan, in his book *Five Lessons*, has students begin with making a half swing with a seven iron. These small, controlled movements set the foundation for the full swing. Remember, wax on/wax off.

Center

Studies show that all movement initiates from the center, the "core" of the body, and moves out into the extremities; the physical center of your body is what Joe Pilates called "the powerhouse," that place from which true power arises. A strong and flexible torso is an extremely powerful tool since the quality of your swing begins at your center. Weakness in the core is the cause of many swing faults and a set up for injury.

Gaining strength and flexibility in the core can protect your lower back, hips and shoulders from pain and injury. To be deeply connected to your center is to bring all of your awareness and attention into focus, centering your mind and emotions and aligning them with your body.

Precision

Precision is focusing attention on each detail of the movement, with the intent of performing that movement perfectly and accurately. When attention is on

CENTER PLAY

Dr. Pink was a student in one of my first Pilates for Golf presentations. About ten days after that presentation, a very elated Dr. Pink was waiting for me outside of class so he could thank me and tell me how his golf game had improved.

"This stuff is amazing," he said. "I'm getting 25 yards more off the tee and on the fairway! And the biggest difference is that I used to play out here"—he stood with his arms spread out wide—"and now, I am playing from here"—he put his palms together in front of his powerhouse.

Dr. Pink had learned how to play from his center.

precision, golfers learn how to stay on their swing plane. Learning to move with precision is one of the keys to accuracy in golf.

Fluidity

The best movement is fluid. Imagine an NBA basketball player charging to the net. He winds his way through the maze of defensive players, charges to the net, and knows exactly when and how to jump and release the ball. The same is true when watching very good golfers—they make it look so effortless. Practicing fluidity in movement also gives golfers a heightened sense of swing tempo. Fluid movement allows elastic energy (power) to build and release throughout the swing. The more fluid the movement, the greater the transfer of powerful energy through the system.

Imagination

Imagery synchronizes the mind and the body to shape movement, whether for an exercise or a golf swing. Visualizing the movement you want to create increases internal awareness and neuromuscular control. Imagine swinging freely.

Body Wisdom

Your body has a language of its own: sensation. You might experience it as a "hunch" or a "gut feeling." Have you ever set up for a shot but it just didn't "feel" right? That's your body wisdom talking to you. Body wisdom is often overlooked and underutilized but it can keep you out of pain, free from injury and moving in the right direction. Listen to your instincts, get a feel for movement and you'll be surprised by what your body-mind already knows. We have all had the experience of becoming frustrated with our game. Eventually we "give up" and stop trying. Then the body wisdom takes over and, suddenly, we return to our natural swing.

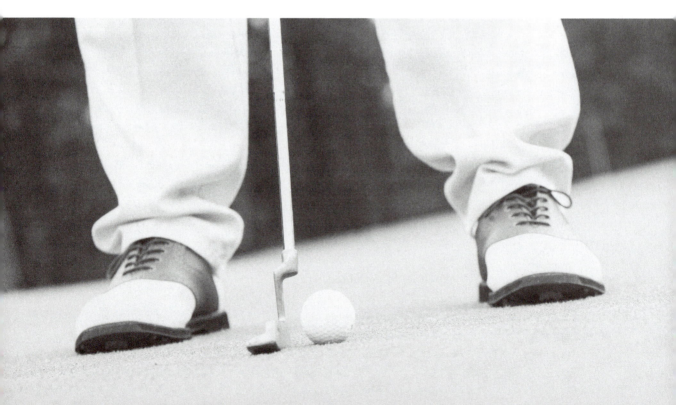

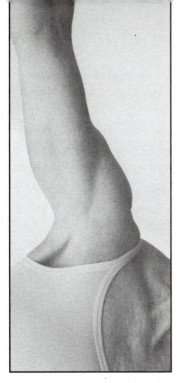

the anatomy of golf

Acquainting yourself with the areas of the body you use when playing golf will enable you to keep them energized yet relaxed while you're at practice or in play. Following is a list of muscle groups and muscle definitions. To keep this section simple, most of the anatomical references are in layperson's terms rather than anatomical ones.

Learning the anatomy of the swing takes some thought and concentration. I want to encourage you to really embrace this part of the program. When you study the list, think of each area and muscle as a piece of a puzzle. If you're interested in studying the exact muscles used, consider picking up *Anatomy of Movement* by Blandine C. Germain or *Physical Golf* by Neil Wolkodoff.

As you begin your study of the anatomy of golf, apply the Pilates principles of concentration and imagination. Notice that when you concentrate on an area of your body, you energize your body-mind con-

nection. Try to imagine how the muscles and tissues are moving as you activate them. This practice will build an inner awareness of playing from your center.

The Core

All movement is generated from the "core," which consists of your neck and torso, from the base of the skull to just below your hip joints. It includes muscles of the abdomen, the back and the pelvic floor. Scientific studies confirm that the deep abdominal muscles are the first to activate in any movement. Gymnasts are a great example of core strength.

Core work is at the heart of every Pilates exercise, developing the muscles that support your spine, hips and shoulders—the areas that are responsible for generating both accuracy and power. The core muscles will help you maintain your spine angle and your balance, which makes staying on your swing plane a cinch. For instance, when you're on an uneven lie, under a tree or have one foot in the bunker, you need to be able to shift your weight and maintain your spine angle all while swinging your club and attempting to remain on your swing plane. By conditioning your core, you'll gain the endurance and strength required for some of these more complex shots. Moreover, because your core muscles support your spine, you'll decrease the threat of injury and golf-related pain to your spine (your lower back especially), your hips and your shoulders.

Think of the core muscles like a girdle. They surround the spine from the front, back, sides and below to support movement in all directions. The muscles are a network of small and large diagonals running in layers, connecting and binding the shoulders, chest and back to the pelvis, hips and legs, wrapping

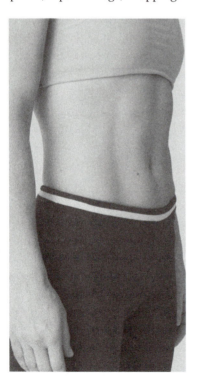

the spine, shoulders and hips like a serape. Other long groups of muscles act like guy wires running up and down the length of the torso. The abdominal and pelvic floor muscles make up what Joseph Pilates called "the Pilates powerhouse." They surround the physical center of gravity in your body. In movement, this center is where true power originates.

The **transverse abdominis** is the deepest of the four abdominal muscles and can become very deconditioned and sleepy. Its fibers run horizontally around your torso, compressing your abdominal wall toward your spine. You can feel it contract when you cough or make a forced exhale. It supports the spine and is very important in maintaining Neutral Spine Angle (see "The Spine" section below) as well as preventing back pain or injury. When golfing, it limits extraneous movement during putting. Learning to activate this core muscle may take some patience, but the value of conditioning it cannot be overstated.

Visualize the **oblique abdominal muscles** as the corset for your waistline. Their fibers run diagonally from your ribs to your hipbones. They are active in side bending and rotating,

and work together to narrow your waistline in toward your spine.

The **rectus abdominis** is the six-pack muscle. The most superficial abdominal muscle, its fibers run vertically from the bottom of the breastbone and ribcage to the pubic bone. Its function is to bend the trunk forward.

The pelvis is shaped like a bowl and every bowl must have a base in order to sit up nicely and be stable. The **pelvic floor muscles** (PFM) are deep, internal muscles attached to the bones in your pelvic cavity; these form the base for the bowl of your pelvis. I call them the elevator muscles because when they contract, they lift up like an elevator. Imagine you are stopping the flow of urine and you'll feel your pelvic floor lifting. The PFM keep your pelvis from wobbling around, giving you better balance and allowing you to maintain neutral spine angle. They are your secret weapon in the putting stroke.

The Spine

Think of your spine as a dynamic, moving pole that bends like the trunk of a tree, allowing you to move in many directions. It can also be like a stable firehouse pole that you

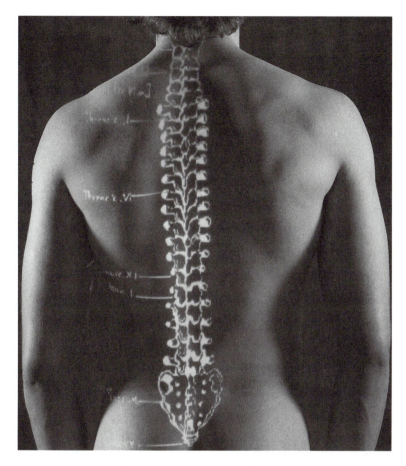

ity and strengthening program, thus establishing the proper spine angle for your game.

In Pilates movement, when your spine is in its naturally curved position, it's called neutral spine. In golf, it's called spine angle. For the purposes of this book, we'll refer to the neutral position of your spine as *neutral spine angle*. Neutral spine angle increases your ability to balance, and movement is at its most efficient, precise and powerful. It's the optimal position from which to swing or putt. Neutral spine angle is also the healthiest position for your back because it naturally places less stress on the muscles, discs and nerves.

Another key movement concept for the spine is its role in rotation. Rotational ability increases when the disc spaces between the vertebrae are decompressed. When the disc spaces are open and mobile, rotation comes easily and with no trauma or pressure to the discs. When in neutral spine angle, the disc spaces are protected *and* rotation is optimal.

The **abdominal core muscles** (see "The Core" above) support the spine from the front of the body.

Several other muscles move and support the spine in golf.

can move around. The spine is at the center of the core and is at the heart of all Pilates-for-golf exercises because it's responsible for so much of what happens within a golf stroke. Moreover, with proper conditioning, the spine can be free from injury and pain.

The spine is made up of 33 separate segments, called vertebra, that originate at the base of the skull and extend to your tailbone. Flat, gel-like discs act as spacers between the verte-

brae. The shape of the vertebral segments in your neck and your lumbar area is designed to form a natural, slightly concave curve and allows for a great deal of movement. The shape and function of the mid-back or thoracic region is different and permits much less spinal movement.

There are three natural curves in the spine, and the proper spine angle for golf is predicated on them. Your goal is to restore the natural curves of your spine through this flexibil-

The **erector spinae** muscles run the length of your spine, from your lumbar spine to your cervical spine. They are active in keeping your spine erect and supported from the back. When your erectors and your core are activated at the same time, we call it "sandwiching the spine," creating simultaneous support from the front and the back.

The **latissimus dorsi** (or "lat") and **trapezius** (or "trap") are large back muscles that act upon the shoulder blades and can be used to enhance the integrity of the shoulder joint and maintain neutral posture. The latissimus dorsi is the widest muscle in your back and connects at the crest of your hips, into connective tissue, at your spine in the mid-torso area, and some of your lower ribs. It wraps around the sides of the body and then twists to attach to your inner upper arm. It pulls your arm back behind you, into your side and rotates it inward, toward your belly.

The large, diamond-shaped trapezius connects your shoulder blade, spine and the part of your shoulder joint that is close to your arm; it's divided into two parts. The fibers of the *upper trap* elevate your shoulder blades; the upper trap tends to be tight. The *lower trap* pulls your shoulder blades down and tends to be weak.

The **quadaratu lumborum** is the "hip hiker" muscle, which hikes the hip upward and is active in side-bending.

The Shoulders and Arms

Your shoulder joint is made up of your shoulder blade, collarbone and the bone of your upper arm. Movement and support for your shoulder joint comes from a complex blend of large and small muscles—the smaller muscles are close to the bones while the larger ones are more superficial. It's important to note that some of the muscles connect the shoulder joint to the chest, the neck and the back. Therefore, if your shoulder has limited mobility, any movement of your arm may affect the other areas. Common imbalances in the muscles of the shoulder joint are often the cause of swing problems.

The muscles of the arm attach to the shoulder blade, the front ribcage and the bone of the upper arm. Due to the design of the shoulder joint, the arm can move easily and in many directions.

The **serratus anterior** attaches your shoulder blade to your ribcage, pulling it down and wide on your back (think football player shoulders). To feel the muscles contract, stand with your arms extended in front of you, palms on a wall. Press your palms into the wall and be aware of the muscle contraction behind and below your armpits. Keeping your shoulder blades down and wide gives the

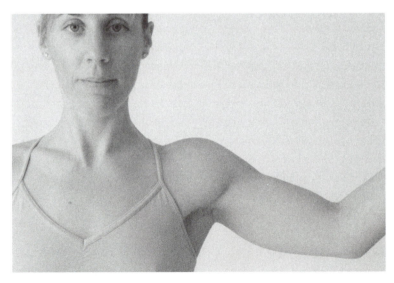

joint integrity and protects the shoulder joint from strains or tears. The serratus tend to be weak.

The **levator scapula** and **rhomboids** are smaller muscles that move your shoulder blades. The levator connects your shoulder blade to your neck and tends to be tight.

The large, diamond-shaped **trapezius** connects your shoulder blade, spine and the part of your shoulder joint that is close to your arm. It's divided into two parts. The fibers of the *upper trap* elevate your shoulder blades; the upper trap tends to be tight. The *lower trap* pulls your shoulder blades down and tends to be weak.

The **rotator cuff** muscles are small and close to the shoulder joint. They rotate the arm inward (toward your belly) and outward (toward your back), and lift the arm out to the side.

The large and superficial **pectoralis major** is one of your chest muscles. It connects at your collarbone, your breastbone and your upper arm.

A smaller muscle called the **teres major** connects your shoulder blade to your arm; like the lat, it pulls your arm back behind you, into your side and rotates it inward, toward your belly.

Your **deltoids** are the "cap" on the top of your shoulder. They connect the shoulder blade, the collarbone and the arm, and lift the arm forward, to the side and backward, depending on which part of it is active.

The **biceps** are connected at your shoulder joint and your forearm. When they contract, they bend your elbow.

The **triceps** connect the back of the shoulder joint, the upper arm and the forearm. When they're active, they straighten the elbow.

The forearm is unique in that it consists of two bones that spiral around one another. Imagine the movement of jiggling a doorknob, allowing our palm to face upward (holding a bowl of soup) then downward; several small muscles with complicated names shape these movements. Another group of muscles has the job of moving the wrists and fingers for wrist cock and for grasping the club.

Some cues for the shoulders and arms:
- Surrender your shoulders down your back.
- Allow your shoulders and arms to be relaxed yet stimulated.
- Soften your upper trapezius by feeling the weight of

your shoulder blades fall down your back.

The Hips and Legs
Your hips are the connection between your lower body and your core, and transfer energy to and from your core. Weight shift, rotation and balance all rely on a smooth transfer of power through your hips. There are six muscles deep in the hip joint that connect the upper thigh (femur) to the pelvis; together, they rotate the femur outward, toward your back. These muscles provide a stable foundation that allows you to stand at address, retrieve your ball from the hole, and engage in all other phases of the game.

The **piriformis**, which connects the sacrum (the bony triangle at the base of the pelvis) to the femur, is one of the six deep rotators that requires special attention from golfers. The piriformis lies close to the sciatic nerve and can affect the nerve when the musculature of the hip joint is not properly balanced.

The **psoas** connects the femur to the lower lumbar spine and is active in lifting the knee toward the chest. It's also active in side-bending. Imbalances in the psoas are common and can lead to discomfort and pain in the groin and lower back during and after golf.

There are three gluteal (buttocks) muscles that support and move your hip. The largest is the **gluteus maximus**, which forms the roundness of your buttock; it connects the pelvis and the leg, extends the femur backward and rotates the pelvis. The other two gluteal muscles are on the outside of your hip joint: the **gluteus minimus** and **medius** lift the leg sideways and are very important in stabilizing the hip joint. Weakness in these two muscles can be a major cause of hip sway.

Other muscles that connect the leg to the pelvis are the large muscles of the thigh: the **quadriceps** group and the **hamstring** group. The *rectus femoris* is the part of the quadriceps group that moves both the hip and the knee; it lifts the femur toward the chest and straightens the leg at the knee. The hamstring group connects the pelvis to the lower leg, crossing the knee. It extends the thigh backward and bends the knee, and acts as a powerful hip rotator during the swing. Together, these muscles are very important in "staying down" in your stance. Weakness in these muscles results in standing up or

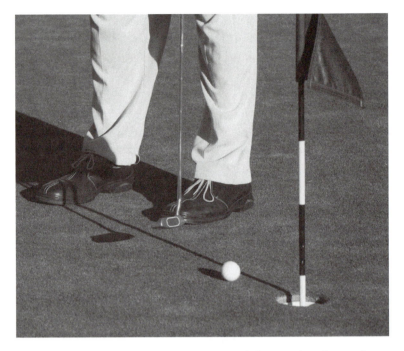

dipping down in the swing.

The **adductor** group connects the pelvis at the inner thigh. When in your stance, it facilitates weight shift by pulling your pelvis in the direction of your standing leg. It's often tight and weak, contributing to hip imbalances.

Finally, the **tensor fascia latae**, or TFL, connects the pelvis to the leg via a band of connective tissue often referred to as the IT band, or iliotibial band. The TFL acts in a number of different movements, but we are mostly concerned with its ability to rotate the femur internally (imagine turning your kneecaps inward to touch one another). Tightness in the TFL limits the rotation of the pelvis

toward the standing leg in the backswing and toward the standing leg in the follow-through.

Cues for the hips/pelvis:

- Shift your hips and your weight from leg to leg by pressing off of the ground. Feel for the inner and outer thigh muscles.
- Shift your weight and rotate side to side and notice how your pelvis rotates around your standing leg.

The Feet and Ankles

Your feet and ankles provide a platform upon which the rest of your body is stacked and balanced. They provide a firm foundation during all phases of the golf stroke. During weight shift, 70 to 90 percent of your weight is transferred to one foot and leg. This is accomplished in part by pushing into the ground to activate muscles. You are essentially balancing most of your weight on one leg while pivoting your hips and coiling your upper body over that leg. Your standing leg becomes the foundation for the rest of your swing movement.

The ability to be well connected to the ground through the feet and ankles is paramount to good weight shift (which generates power for the swing) and to maintaining balance (which keeps you on your swing plane). If the feet and ankles are not adequately conditioned, the ability to generate power from the ground through the core is limited.

There are numerous muscles and movements in the lower leg. For golf, we'll focus on the calf muscles: the **gastrocnemius** and the **soleus**. These two muscles flex the ankle and are active in walking. Point your toes and you'll feel them. Tight muscles and tendons in the back of the lower leg restrict the ability of the ankle to bend (think the opposite of pointing your toes); restricted movement of the ankles affects the ability to get into and hold the address position.

The deeper of the two muscles is the soleus, which connects the two bones of the lower leg to the heel via the Achilles tendon. The more superficial gastrocnemius connects the ankle to the knee, so it does two things: it flexes the ankle like the soleus and bends the knee as well.

Both the gastrocnemius and soleus flex on the take-away side to shift the weight and to move the lower leg and foot into the end position. The muscles of the lower leg are also active in maintaining balance throughout the swing.

Cues for the feet:
- Notice how your feet connect to the ground. Ground yourself into your feet, allowing your center of gravity to move from your head (thinking) to your core (sensing).

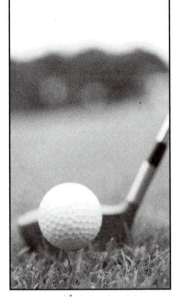

the big picture

When you shift your focus from movement mechanics to swing mechanics, you heighten your body awareness, one of the elements of the body-mind connection. When you play with body awareness, you play the game from the inside out. Most people gain an entirely new perspective on their game. Through awareness and consistency, your body-mind equipment becomes finely tuned for the game. This section will take you through the swing sequence so that you can see the whole movement picture.

At Address

The address position gives you the optimal base for your golf swing. Your *core abdominal muscles* and *back muscles* sandwich your spine to maintain the neutral spine angle; your *hamstrings* and *buttocks* support you from below. Your arms are active, yet relaxed, with the *triceps* gently engaged to straighten the arms. Stability of the pelvis and spine during the golf swing is one of the keys to developing accuracy.

The Backswing

The purpose of your backswing is to create the coil of elastic energy for release on your downswing. Think of it as stretching back the band on a slingshot before releasing it. Your goal is to make a nice, long arc with your arms, which puts you into position for the optimal club-head speed. The *forearm muscles* maintain the grip of the club. Your *leg muscles* initiate the slide of your hips to the take-away side; the *adductors* on the take-away side initiate weight shift. The *hamstrings* rotate the hips, and the *core oblique abdominals* and the *back muscles* on the take-away side rotate the pelvis. The *muscles in the back and the rear of the shoulder* on the take-away side turn the torso and shoulders, while the *deltoids* on the take-away side lift the arms up and back. *Biceps* on the take-away side bend the take-away elbow. *Rotator cuff muscles* on the take-away side rotate the arm and help to maintain shoulder position; the *lower traps* also keep the shoulders in position. In your backswing, your *pectoralis major* is stretched out.

The Downswing

This is the release of the elastic coil. Your *adductors* on the front side initiate weight shift while your *feet and legs* initiate the slide of your hips to the front leg and begin rotation. The *TFL* and *gluteus minimus* on the front side rotate the hips as your *core oblique abdominals* rotate your torso. Your "*hip hiker*" *muscle* begins the torso side-bending movement. Your shoulders follow, with the *pectoralis* drawing the back arm down. Your *shoulders* rotate your arms and your *forearms*

begin to roll your wrists; the *triceps* keeps the front arm straight and the *lower traps* are active in maintaining shoulder position. The *pectoralis* pulls the arm through, helping to bring your take-away-side arm back down and through impact.

At Impact

The *spinal muscles* are very active during impact; the *abdominal core* stabilizes the spine. Your *feet and legs* continue with the weight shift and your core (particularly the *obliques*) continues with the hip rotation. The "*hip hiker*" *muscle* is still active in side-bending. The *pectoralis* and *shoulders* still remain active, with the *pectoralis* on the take-away side continuing the club's movement. The *obliques* draw the take-away shoulder into posi-

tion. The *rotator cuff muscles* on both sides rotate the arms and keep the shoulders in position; the *latissimus* on the take-away side also rotates the arm. The *erector spinae* and *lat* are active in the rotation of the spine. The

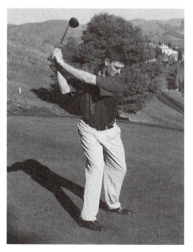

The Backswing

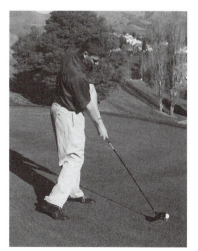

At Impact

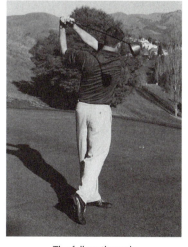

The follow-through

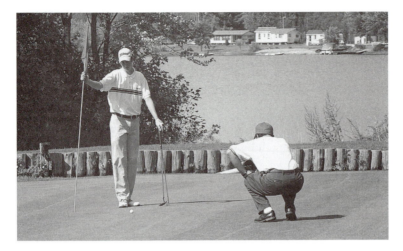

triceps straighten the arms and the *forearms* remain active in wrist release. The *adductors, TFL* and *gluteus minimus* continue their action from the downswing into follow-through.

Follow-through

The follow-through continues the path of the body through the hitting plane and safely slows the tremendous momentum of the swing. Weight shift and rotation is completed by the *back, hamstrings* and *gluteus muscles.* The torso and arms continue mostly due to momentum; the *back* and *rear shoulders* draw the arms around and up (the *lower traps* can remain engaged to maintain shoulder position). In some cases, the back (*erector spinae*) goes into hyperextension. The *abdominal*

core and erector spinae rotate and stabilize, taking the upright finish into neutral spine angle. The *rotator cuff muscle* on the take-away side protects the shoulder joint from overrotating, while the rotator cuff muscles on the front side rotate the arm. The *forearms* remain active to grip the club.

Putting

The putting stance, grip and arm positions vary according to each golfer's needs. The elements that create a solid putting stroke, however, are the same for every golfer. The ability to remain balanced over your feet requires strong stance muscles. The pendulum-type stroke requires strong pelvic floor muscles, all of the abdominal muscles, as well as the erector spinae muscles.

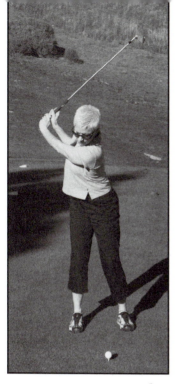

healthy body, healthy golf

During my very first golf lesson, especially with my athletic background, I was incredulous that I was doing so poorly swinging the club, attempting to hit the ball, and trying to figure out what I was supposed to be doing. "It feels so awkward!" I said to my pro. "That's because golf is not a natural movement," he replied.

That was it—the match that lit the fire. The idea that the golf swing is not a natural movement intrigued me and sparked a million movement questions, the foremost being: If a golf swing is not a natural movement, what is it doing to our bodies?

It's not surprising that many golfers are playing with some kind of pain. The physical demands of golf are highly specialized and many golfers simply don't have the flexibility, strength or stamina to uphold the precise and repetitive movements. Because the golf swing isn't a natural movement, there are plenty of opportunities for

poor biomechanics, which means less-than-optimal movement patterns that often lead to pain and/or injuries.

In general, novice golfers try to repeat this unnatural movement precisely, numerous times over the course of four hours! Most golfers haven't built the physical or mental endurance to last the duration of their play. When there's a lack of stamina, the body and mind begin to break down from fatigue. When the system begins to fatigue, it starts to compensate. Compensation changes the swing pattern because when your golfing muscles fatigue, different muscles begin to take over. Ben

Hogan, in his book *Five Lessons*, likens this situation to watching a Western movie: "The way the parts of the body function in the golf swing is, in fact, not unlike a Western movie with heroes and villains: if you set it up so that the good guys take over, the bad guys can't."

When compensation takes place, different muscles (villains) take over, kind of like using the spare tire on your car. Using these spare muscles causes changes in your swing, thereby altering your swing arc. Spare muscles are not endurance muscles—they fatigue quickly and thus are only good for a short time.

Once compensation sets in, we try harder to "find" our swing again . . . but we end up compensating more. At this point, we're playing with a "compensation swing." If we continue to play with the compensation swing, we end up grooving the compensation swing into our muscle memory. For the higher-handicap golfer, injuries often occur once the system has defaulted into a compensation pattern. The lower-handicap golfer's injuries are more likely to stem from repetitive movement and over-stretching of soft tissue.

Golf-specific conditioning prevents injury by training the body to move efficiently and effectively, thereby increasing endurance and allowing us to play with our "true" swing pat-tern (heroes) throughout the entire game.

If you want to improve your golf game and stay pain-free, you need to train yourself as an athlete. Athletes engage in con-ditioning programs to develop the physical and mental prowess necessary for their game, as well as to prevent injury and pain. Many golfers find that they can return to the demands of tournament play after undertaking a conditioning program; those who had previ-ously given up playing two to three days in a row are now playing strong and feeling great at the end of the tournament. The golf-specific training in this book will reduce your risk of injury and decrease the event of pain during and after your game.

Where Does It Hurt?

To play a great game, you must achieve full range of motion, along with the ability to main-tain posture and balance while moving quickly and powerfully. If your joints are not fully functional with a balance of flexibility and strength, you run the risk of injury or pain. Statistics show that about 53 percent of male golfers and 45 percent of female golfers play with some kind of pain. Higher-handicap golfers make mistakes due to poor skill levels that compromise their body biomechanics. This can be exacerbated by "excessive use of force," better known as trying to kill the ball. As you practice the exercises in this book, you'll train your body and mind to create efficient and effective movement so that excessive force is replaced by fluidity and finesse. In addition, you'll pro-tect your joints from the wear and tear of the unnatural golf movement.

The most common complaint among golfers is chronic lower back pain, particularly on the take-away side. It's not unusual for players to finish in a back-bend, hyperextending into a backward "C." Many players learned to finish this way and don't have problems related to this position. However, if you suffer from lower back tension or pain related to golf and you finish with a "C" curve, you might want to work with your pro to learn to finish with a longer, more neutral spine position.

Many golfers stop playing due to lower back pain, while others play anyway, taking extra doses of anti-inflammatory drugs to get through the round. Limited range of motion in the

---

FUEL THE FIRE

Your cardiovascular system oxygenates your blood and feeds your brain. Optimal cardiovascular health increases endurance, decreases tension and mental stress, and im-proves the overall level of play. If you'd like more information about cardiovascular training, contact the American Council on Exercise: www.ace.org.

hip area can cause stress to the area above the hip, generally the lower back, and at the knee. Most of the time, lower back discomfort can be alleviated through conditioning. With more information about the mechanics of the spine and the muscles that support it, as well as a good conditioning program, many golfers have been able play better with little or no discomfort.

The shoulders, wrists and elbows are also typical sites of injury or chronic pain. High-handicap golfers, beginning golfers and women are especially prone to wrist and elbow injuries. The Pilates stretches and exercises will build both strength and flexibility into the shoulders, forearms and wrists. Additionally, golfing from the core will decrease the

tendency to overuse the arms and hands, thereby reducing the risk of injury and chronic discomfort from overuse.

Golfers may suffer from plantar fasciitis, inflammation of the connective tissue that results in pain through the heel and arch of the foot. Ankle injuries are not common, but tightness in the muscles and tendons of the lower leg, such as the Achilles tendon, do affect the flexibility and mobility of the ankle joint. Exercises for the feet and ankles are aimed at maintaining strength and flexibility in the muscles of the lower leg that attach to the bones of the heels and ankles, as well as the soft connective tissues and muscles that support the arch of the foot.

If you live with chronic pain or have suffered an injury, I rec-

SWING FAULTS

One of the most common swing faults is failure to shift the weight onto the front leg at impact and follow-through, which means most of the weight remains on the back leg. In this case, when the upper body continues into the follow-through, the lower spine moves into a reverse "C" curvature, compressing the lower lumbar area. This reverse pivot position is one of the most damaging to the lower back. It's generally caused by weakness and inflexibility in the hips and legs.

ommend you see a good physical therapist (PT) prior to beginning this program. If you can, find a PT who specializes in sports medicine. Chances are, a PT will understand the Pilates philosophy and can help you modify your *Golfer's Guide* program for your needs. You might also consider training with a Pilates for Golf Coach™ instructor. These golf-conditioning specialists are trained in assessment skills and can tailor a program specifically for your needs. Find a list of trained PFGCoach™ instructors on page 136.

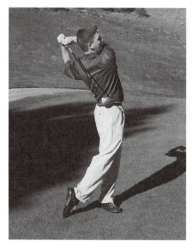

Incorrect follow-through: the lower spine is in a reverse "C"

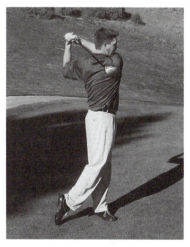

Correct follow-through: longer, more neutral spine position

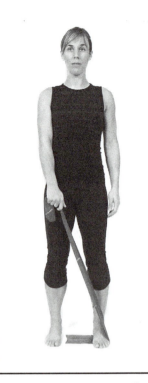

before you begin

In addition to generating motivation, preparing yourself physically and mentally will help you stay committed to your new exercise program. The following tips will give you a solid foundation from which to start your journey to a better body and a better game.

A Successful Startup

As with any exercise regimen, you must speak with your doctor before beginning this program. If you have lower back, neck, shoulder or other problems that are exacerbated by exercise, you should seek advice from a physician, physical therapist or health practitioner prior to undertaking this program. Once you have been released from care, you may begin.

Creating the Space

Part of developing a regular practice is creating a space that's set aside especially for your workouts. Make the space invit-ing and personal so you look forward to spending time in it. Make sure the surface of the floor is comfortable for sitting and lying by keeping it clean and soft, yet supportive. A yoga mat is a perfect choice because it defines your area nicely and you can roll it up when you're not using it. If you have a tile or other hard surface, try placing a small throw rug under your yoga mat.

Toys and Equipment

There's not much equipment required to do *The Golfer's Guide to Pilates* programs. However, some items are helpful to have, and the foam roller is integral to your flexibility and balance training.

A **small throw pillow** or **towel** will help with proper alignment and is useful for stretching and added support.

A wide variety of **yoga mats** are available nowadays. I recommend Gaiam mats, which can be found at Whole Foods Markets or ordered online at www.gaiam.com. My personal favorite, the Eco Mat, is made from natural fibers, which makes it non-slip as well as washable; it's available at www.greenyoga.com.

Elastic exercise bands come in a variety of tensions and are used to build strength and flexi-

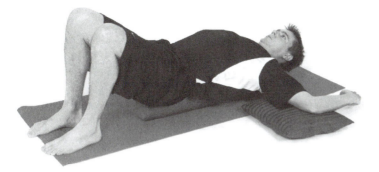

Dylan uses a small pillow for a little added support in this chest release exercise.

bility. They're a common tool for rehabilitating injuries.

Although **balance balls** are known primarily for building balance and conditioning the core muscles, *The Golfer's Guide to Pilates* uses it for an important breathing exercise.

The Essentials programs do not require anything other than space, a mat and your patience. The other programs in this book utilize a **foam roller**, which release tight muscles, are great stretching devices and are incredible balance tools. Release work, a form of self-massage, restores the resilience of the connective tissues, or myofascial tissue, increasing range of motion and the ability of your muscles to contract fully and efficiently. Since performing release work with a roller deeply affects the soft tissues, it can be a bit uncomfortable for the first few weeks. With consistent roller work, the tissues become supple and healthy once more, and the discomfort will decrease (don't be surprised if you become addicted to it). Learning the rolling routine feels a little awkward at first, but once you get the hang of it, the routine is a quick and effective way to enhance your body and your game.

I believe everyone should own at least one roller: they're inexpensive, don't take up much space, and are one of the best investments you can make to improve your body and your game. All of my students use foam rollers, and have at least one at home and one for travel; some of my students travel with an extra golf bag just so they can pack their foam roller in it. Rollers are widely available but the quality does vary. You can order good-quality foam rollers from OPTP physical therapy products at www.optp.com.

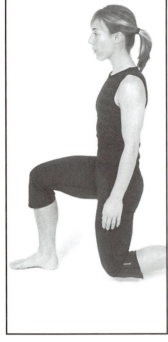

key pilates concepts

You've probably gotten the idea that there's much more to the Pilates Method than just a bunch of exercises. In fact, learning the Pilates Method of movement is like golf in that it has its own language and concepts that drive each exercise. Here I have compiled a list of key Pilates movement concepts to help you make the most of each exercise.

These mind-body concepts make use of your imagination to help you maintain the connection between your mind and your body for optimal performance and to assist you in maintaining good form throughout your movements. And remember: engaging and activating muscles with only as much effort as necessary to get the job done (basically, moving with as little effort as possible) will help you stay relaxed and fluid in your movements.

Neutral spine angle

Your spine has three natural curves at the neck, mid-back and lower back. The spine is healthiest when its curves are elongated, or lengthened, rather that compressed and exaggerated. When the spinal curves are in the lengthened, natural position, they're in what's called neutral spine angle. Neutral spine angle places your spine in the proper spine angle for golf. Neutral spine angle creates space for the discs, protecting them from the shearing force of rotation. It also elongates the

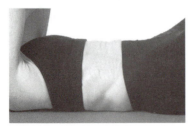

Incorrect Neutral Spine: Too Flat

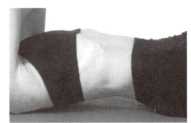

Incorrect Neutral Spine: Too Arched

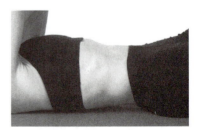

Correct Neutral Spine

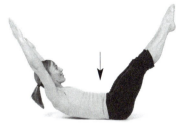

The powerhouse

spine, allowing for greater rotation, increased club-head speed and greater power through the swing. See "Primer on Pilates Positions" on page 38 for information on how to sit and stand with neutral spine angle.

The Powerhouse

The powerhouse muscles are your abdominal and pelvic floor muscles. To engage your powerhouse muscles, imagine lifting your belly in and up as if an imaginary corset were being tightened around your midsection. Your pelvic floor and abdominal muscles engage, creating a "hollowing" of the lower abdomen.

Navel to Spine

Navel to spine is an imagery cue that, when practiced properly, engages the deepest layer of abdominal muscles, the transverse abdominis (TVA). When the TVA is strong, it acts like a corset around the sides and front of the torso from the ribcage to the pelvis. The TVA compresses the abdomen toward the spine, providing support from the front and sides. To feel the navel-to-spine sensation, imagine zipping up a pair of jeans that's too small for you: exhale and begin pulling your belly in and up in a scooping motion toward the spine.

Shoulders into Back Pockets

Strengthening the muscles that pull the shoulder blades down and wide keeps the shoulders strong and allows for full range of motion. Strong and flexible shoulders permit greater shoulder turn and increase ability to direct power from the core to the club. The imagery cue "draw your shoulders down your spine and into your back pockets" provides the mental and physical connection to the muscles in the upper body that need strengthening and stretching.

A SOLID FOUNDATION

The stance is the foundation for the entire swing—the foundation from which you move—so when your core is strong, your stance is strong. When your ankles, legs, buttocks, back and abs have the right combination of strength and flexibility, they can support weight shift and rotation without losing your spine angle or your swing arc.

Practice your stance with neutral spine angle in the mirror. Find the three natural curves of the spine. Use your powerhouse muscles to lengthen the spine and then sandwich it front and back. Try relaxing, but staying active, with your sandwich muscles. Then take it to the range.

Sandwich Your Spine

When you draw on the powerhouse to support the spine from the front and the "shoulders into your back pockets" muscles to support the spine from the back, you create a supporting "sandwich" for the spine.

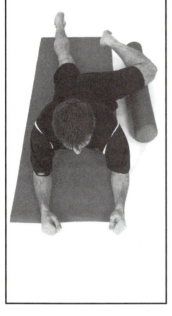

primer on pilates positions

Positioning yourself properly for each exercise is like going through the set-up before you swing. It's the mental and physical preparation for your movement. Each Pilates exercise arises from one of the following positions.

On Your Back with Neutral Spine Angle

Lie on your back with your knees bent and arms extended along your sides, palms down. Place your feet flat on the floor, lining up your hips, knees and feet.

Relax your neck, letting your chin drop toward the floor. Imagine you are making a dou-

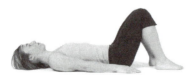

On your back with neutral spine angle

ble chin and feel the curve of your neck lengthen.

Next, relax your ribcage and chest, letting the area around your shoulder blades soften into the floor. Imagine your back spreading out like a pancake on a griddle, growing wider and fuller. Try to touch your back lower ribs onto the floor.

Finally, imagine your belly is filled with water. Tilt your pelvis as if to spill the water between your legs; your lower back will arch away from the floor. Then tilt your pelvis in the opposite direction as if to spill the water toward your

head; your lower back will flatten to the floor. Arch and flatten 10 times and then come to rest in a neutral position somewhere between arched and flattened. You should have just enough space for two fingertips to slide easily between your lower back and the floor.

Knees to Ceiling with Neutral Spine Angle

Begin on your back in neutral spine angle. On an exhale, lift the right foot off the floor so that the right knee cap is pointing directly to the ceiling, then lift the left knee cap toward the

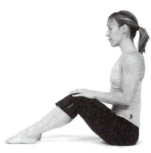

Sitting with neutral spine angle

ceiling. Maintain the neutral position of your pelvis with both knees to the ceiling.

Peel-Up Position

Begin in Knees to Ceiling position. On an exhale, imagine you are peeling your spine off the floor, beginning with your neck. Roll your chin toward your chest, your chest toward your ribcage and glide your ribcage toward your pelvis until just the bottom edge of your shoulder blades are in contact with the floor. Your lower back will gently contact the floor in this position.

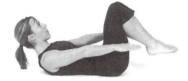

Peel-Up position

Side-lying with Neutral Spine Angle

Begin on your back in neutral spine angle. Maintain the natural curves of your spine while you roll onto your right side. Stack your left hip on top of your right and extend your legs, sliding them forward a few inches. Place your right elbow on the floor exactly beneath your right shoulder, press your forearm into the ground, lift your hips off the floor and press

your right shoulder away from your right ear. Place your left hand on the floor in front of you like a kickstand on a bicycle.

Lift your ribcage toward the ceiling to keep your neutral spine angle. Try to avoid letting your front ribs splay forward.

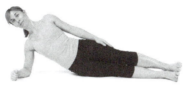

Side-lying with neutral spine angle

Sitting with Neutral Spine Angle

Sit on top of your "sitting bones," the pointy bones in your buttocks that feel like two little speed bumps. Create a small curve in your lower back by sitting up tall, lengthening your spine by reaching the top of your head to the ceiling; try to increase the space between your ribcage and your pelvis.

Lengthen your neck by making a slight double chin. Pull your front ribs in and up as you draw your shoulder blades down your back.

Tip: If you're unable to sit up without collapsing forward, wedge a prop such as a rolled-up towel or a small pillow under the back half of your buttocks for support.

Hands and Knees with Neutral Spine Angle

Come on to your hands and knees. Place your hands directly beneath your shoulders and your knees directly beneath your hips. Lengthen your spine from your head to your tailbone.

To find the three natural curves of your spine:

Lengthen your neck so your forehead is parallel to the floor. Look at one spot on the floor to keep your head in the correct position.

Draw your shoulders down and wide on your back. Let them be broad like a football player's shoulders. Lengthen the space between your shoulder blades.

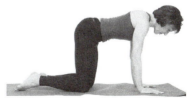

Hands and Knees
with neutral spine angle

Create a small curve in your lower lumbar area. It may feel like your tailbone is sticking up in the air.

Belly-Down with Neutral Spine Angle

Lie on your belly with your arms extended along your sides, your fingertips reaching for your toes. Place your forehead on the floor to keep the curve of your neck long.

Allow your lower back to relax: Imagine it is lengthening as your hip bones and pubic bone sink toward the floor. Keep your hip joints moving

Belly-Down with neutral spine angle

toward the floor.

Lift the abdominal wall and the pelvic floor without changing the position of your pelvis.

Tip: Avoid overarching your lower back in this position—use your abdominals and modify your movements if you experience back discomfort.

Standing with Neutral Spine Angle

You can place a dowel (or even a driver, if you prefer) behind your back to check for neutral spine angle in standing.

Have a friend hold a dowel or club up to your spine. The back of your head, your midback and your sacrum (the bony triangle at the base of your spine) should touch the club.

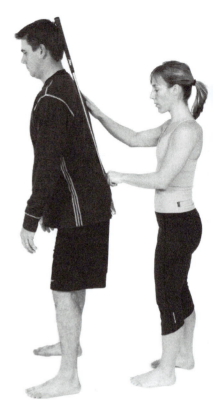

Louise helps Dylan find neutral spine.

part two:
the
programs

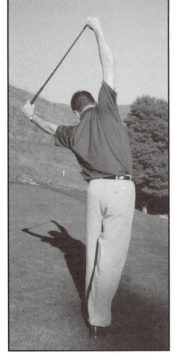

get into the swing

In this section you'll find ten different golf conditioning programs. The first two weeks of your new regimen begins with the Flexibility First Program. The Essentials Program has three levels and is a full-body workout that will integrate your body-mind for the movement of golf. Anyone with good overall health can begin the Flexibility First and the Essentials Level 1 Program.

Whether you are new to the Pilates concepts or have some Pilates background, learn the Essentials Level 1 Program first. Once you get to know the Essentials programs, you can easily practice at home, at the gym and even when you're traveling. It's a great overall program that will give you a solid handle on the fundamental movements for golf. If you want to make additional improvements, the Specialty Programs address common imbalances golfers may have, such as hip sway, poor rotation and limited shoulder turn.

Play It Safe

No matter what level you're at, work at your own pace and integrate the Pilates mind/body principles and the Principles of Power (page 18) into each exercise.

It's also more important to perform exercises properly rather than to do all the repetitions of any exercise; if you find yourself losing your form, either rest for a moment and start again, or just move on to the next exercise. You may find some exercises surprisingly easy and others especially challenging. Your strength and stamina will increase with consistency. If at any time you feel pain or discomfort during a movement, especially in the neck and lower back, use a modification or stop the exercise until you gain the stability and strength you need to execute it properly.

Some cues may not make sense to you at first, but as you repeat the exercises, you'll begin to develop a feel for the more subtle movements and cues. Keep the book handy, as you'll need to refer to it frequently when you are learning new movements.

Commitment and Consistency

A successful program is built upon consistency and commitment over a length of time. Here are some ideas to keep you on track and focused on your ultimate goal of healthy, powerful golf:

- Make an appointment with yourself. Create a workout schedule for yourself and write your name in your appointment book. Be sure to include time for your cardiovascular training.
- The Flexibility First and Essentials Level 1 workouts begin with three days per week. Try to schedule your workouts so they are spaced equally throughout the week. The Essentials need to be practiced consistently in order to build the body memory of the exercises, so large spaces of time between practice will impair your forward momentum.
- If you skip a workout or a few in a row, just pick up and start again. Visualize your program over the period of a year or longer. If you just keep moving forward, one or two missed workouts here and there over time isn't a big deal.

- Don't judge a book by its cover. You probably won't walk away from your workout with your legs shaking and your muscles burning. So if you're accustomed to a workout that gives you the "burn," you may have to overcome the "no pain, no gain" concept before you can appreciate the uniqueness of Pilates work. Give yourself time to get into Level 2 of the Essentials workout and you'll find you are building a different kind of strength from a different kind of workout.

Plan to devote 30–45 minutes of uninterrupted time to each session. Initially, your sessions will address flexibility issues. The Flexibility First and the Essentials Level 1 workouts are germane to the entire program. This is where the wax on/wax off principle is most important. It takes about three to four weeks for your body and mind to learn new ways to move. Once you have memorized the Essentials Level 1, you may adjust the length of time and frequency to fit your schedule. You can do the Flexibility and Essentials every day if you'd like. As you move

forward with your program, you can design your program to include a combination of flexibility and additional exercises to suit your needs within the allotted time you have set aside for your training.

Specialize It

Each of us brings a unique set of strengths and weaknesses to our game. Like a fingerprint, our areas of balance and imbalance show up in the groove of our swing and are reflected in our swing faults. Think of your swing faults like a mirror, giving you clear feedback about those areas of your body-mind that are in good balance and those areas that could use improvement. Your swing faults can guide you in designing a program that is tailored specifically to your needs. The Specialty Programs target the areas where common imbalances occur. They are not meant to be golf-specific programs within themselves, but additional programs to address areas of imbalance. For instance, if you know you want to increase hip rotation, read the Hip Turn Program for a better understanding of how that area affects your game and blend that program into your Essentials program.

flexibility first program
3–5 times per week for 30 minutes

Remember, golf requires balanced and integrated movement. The first step to shaping a strong body capable of generating power is restoring flexibility to the entire system. Our muscles and connective tissues hold our joints together and allow them to move in their unique ways. When there is balance between the muscles, connective tissues and bones of the joints, we enjoy full range of motion at that joint. The joint is flexible and strong; it has the integrity to move properly and protect itself from injury. When our joints and tissues are balanced, they have a harmonious relationship between them, called the "length-tension" relationship.

Strength, power and finesse for golf are reliant upon balanced length-tension relationships in our joints. Inflexibility at any joint upsets the length-tension relationship, decreases joint integrity and degrades movement. The Flexibility First Program uses the foam roller to release muscle and connective tissue and static and active stretches to restore balance to the joints.

You'll be gaining dynamic flexibility throughout the remainder of the program due to the unique quality of the Pilates philosophy; each Pilates exercise has a stretching and strengthening component. Most areas of the body will balance out quickly. As those areas balance out, you can discontinue the static stretching exercises. Then, if an area gets tight again, you'll know how to balance it out with static stretches. However, many golfers have areas of chronic tightness. For example, many men have chronically tight hamstrings. If you find you have some stubborn areas, you may continue to do the static release exercises for that area indefinitely, even as you move forward into the Essentials Program.

Flexibility training requires mindfulness when executing the movements, so your mental training in focused concentration begins with this program. Proper breathing techniques enhance the release process and build the body-mind connection.

The Flexibility First Program will require approximately 30 minutes, at least three times per week, for two to three weeks. This program can be done every day if you are inclined. If you're very inflexible, stay with the program for three weeks. If you're fairly flexible, work with the program for two weeks.

The roller release work can be done anytime, pre- and post-game. The flexibility exercises are best done post-game and in the evening, after play, because the static stretches (ones that you hold for 45 seconds) are sedating to the nervous system.

In Part 4, you'll find the Pre-swing Warm-ups that will best prepare you for the practice range and your game.

flexibility first

FLEXIBILITY FIRST

	61	neck release
	62	spine release
	63	back extension
	64	lat release
	65	soften the buns
	66	IT band release
	67	inner thigh release
	68	calf release
	69	chest release
	70	lower back release
	71	side and forward neck stretch
	77	side-lying shoulder circles
	76	shoulder and chest stretches
	75	wrist flexion stretch
	78	crescent moon
	80	modified swan
	82	lat stretch
	83	split squat stretch
	84	knee over
	85	"hippest" hip stretch

the essentials program level 1
3 times per week for 30 minutes

No matter what your level of conditioning is now, unless you already have a deep understanding of the Pilates Method and functional training movements and principles, everybody begins their study of this program with Level 1 essentials.

Think of Level 1 as the fundamentals. Just like the fundamentals of golf, the fundamentals of golf movement are the foundation from which all other movement will take place. This is the wax on/wax off part of the program.

If you're athletic or have a regular exercise program, you might be tempted to skip over the Level 1 basics, especially because at first they can seem simplistic. However, keep in mind that the Level 1 basics are

the gateway to true power and the only way to get there is by practicing them mindfully.

The Pilates system is unique in that we don't do traditional "sets" and "repetitions." Because the exercises are an integration of muscle systems rather than isolated muscles, they are much more intense in nature.

In the Essentials Level 1 phase, if you can execute 3 to 5 good movements in the beginning, you're doing well. Do not sacrifice your form in order to do more movements or you'll just end up building greater muscle imbalances. If there's a modified version of an exercise, practice the modification first and progress to the full expression of the movement slowly.

Always begin your session with **breathing exercises** (pages 58–60). And since some areas of your body will most likely need flexibility training indefinitely, keep in mind the **flexibility exercises** (pages 71–87) that you feel are most beneficial and do them at the end of whichever Essentials program you are working with. (Hint: The ones you like the least are usually the ones you need the most.)

Plan to spend 10–12 sessions on the Level 1 workout before moving on to Level 2. If you've been inconsistent with your workouts, plan to spend more time on Level 1. You should have an understanding of the movements and be fairly proficient executing them prior to advancing to Level 2.

the essentials program

LEVEL 1

	72	neck turn
	96	the hundred
	97	single-leg stretch
	102	pendulum
	108	leg circles
	73	hand stretch
	86	shoulder circles
	87	external shoulder rotation
	110	side-lying leg circles
	111	up and down
	107	mermaid (modified)
	100	spine twist
	103	ab lift
	89	serratus anterior push-ups (modified)
	112	split squat
	113	standing balance
	114	weight shift
	81	rest pose

the essentials program level 2
3–4 times per week for 40 minutes

Once you have a good working knowledge of the Essentials Level 1 movements and have achieved proper form, build upon that base by adding more challenging exercises and increasing the number of times each exercise is executed. Sessions 10–20 will challenge you to gain stability and strength.

Always begin your session with **breathing exercises** (pages 58–60). And since some areas of your body will most likely need flexibility training indefinitely, keep in mind the **flexibility exercises** (pages 71–87) that you feel are most beneficial and do them at the end of whichever Essentials program you are working with. (Hint: The ones you like the least are usually the ones you need the most.)

Plan to spend about 10 sessions at Level 2. If there are Level 1 exercises that are still challenging due to strength and/or flexibility issues, continue doing those exercises while working on the Level 2 exercises. If you've been inconsistent with your workouts, plan to spend more time on Level 2. You should be fairly proficient at executing the Level 2 exercises prior to advancing to Level 3.

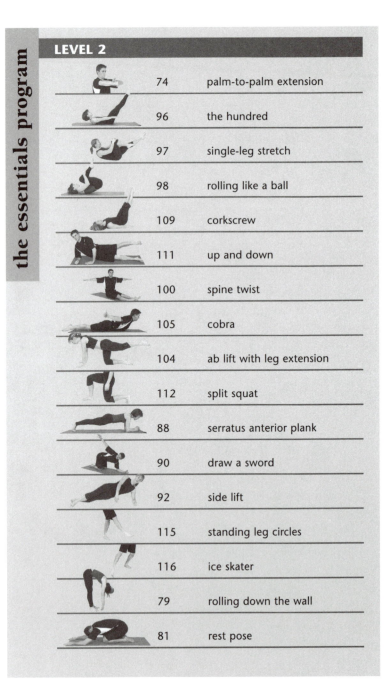

the essentials program

LEVEL 2

	74	palm-to-palm extension
	96	the hundred
	97	single-leg stretch
	98	rolling like a ball
	109	corkscrew
	111	up and down
	100	spine twist
	105	cobra
	104	ab lift with leg extension
	112	split squat
	88	serratus anterior plank
	90	draw a sword
	92	side lift
	115	standing leg circles
	116	ice skater
	79	rolling down the wall
	81	rest pose

the essentials program level 3
3–5 times per week for 40 minutes

Essentials Level 3 movements are whole-body integration exercises that require the solid foundation of Levels 1 and 2 in order to be effective. This level includes the advanced and super-advanced versions of the exercises. You should have at least 30 sessions under your belt to be sure your core is strong and your joints can support these movements.

Always begin your session with **breathing exercises** (pages 58–60). And since some areas of your body will most likely need flexibility training indefinitely, keep in mind the **flexibility exercises** (pages 71–87) that you feel are most beneficial and do them at the end of whichever Essentials program you are working with. (Hint: The ones you like the least are usually the ones you need the most.)

More than likely you will find that a few of the exercises in Levels 1 and 2 still challenge you. As you move on to Level 3, carry the more challenging exercises from the previous levels over to this level and add them to your sessions. It can take up to several months to do some of the exercises properly.

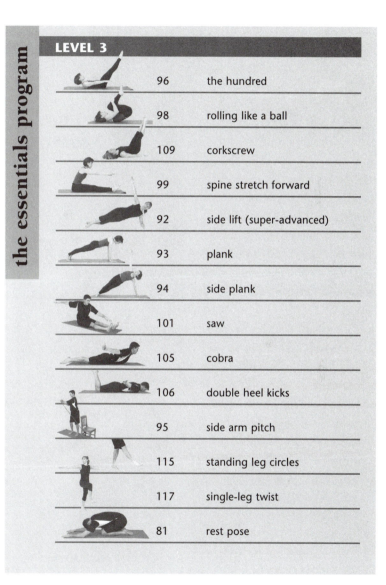

the essentials program

LEVEL 3

	96	the hundred
	98	rolling like a ball
	109	corkscrew
	99	spine stretch forward
	92	side lift (super-advanced)
	93	plank
	94	side plank
	101	saw
	105	cobra
	106	double heel kicks
	95	side arm pitch
	115	standing leg circles
	117	single-leg twist
	81	rest pose

specialty programs
the stance

In golf, each stroke is based upon your set-up position, which includes finding and holding your spine angle throughout your movement. During the swing, the spine has to remain neutral, rotate, bend sideways and in some cases extend backwards while building and releasing the tremendous force of elastic energy. In putting, the spine must stay absolutely still in some areas while allowing controlled movement in others.

Developing strong stance muscles will help you avoid common swing faults like standing up or sitting down in the swing and excessive hip sway. Additionally, strong stance muscles will prevent those faulty movements that so often cause pain and injury to the knees, hips and back.

Initially, you may need to reduce the length of your swing in order to maintain your spine angle, but as you learn to play from your center and become strong enough to hold it, you'll

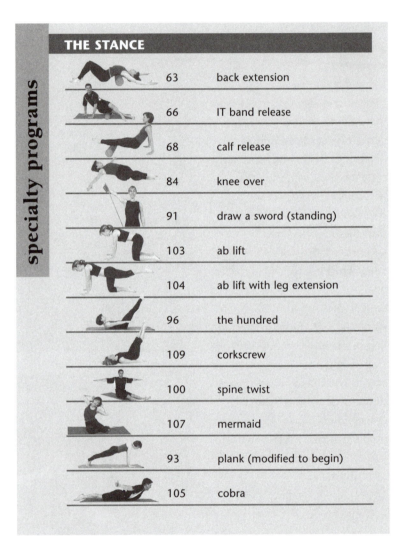

specialty programs		
THE STANCE		
	63	back extension
	66	IT band release
	68	calf release
	84	knee over
	91	draw a sword (standing)
	103	ab lift
	104	ab lift with leg extension
	96	the hundred
	109	corkscrew
	100	spine twist
	107	mermaid
	93	plank (modified to begin)
	105	cobra

find your accuracy improving. From there you can lengthen your swing incrementally. This is the basis for power.

In addition to doing the exercises listed here, do the **flexibility exercises** (pages 71–87) that target your problem areas.

specialty programs
core strength

You can improve the quality of your movement by building awareness of how your musculature supports your spine and how your spine supports your movement. Let the size and depth of your movements be determined by the strength and stability of your spine.

The great thing about the core muscles is that you can activate them anytime, in just about any position. You don't need any special equipment, just your awareness. Some people practice activating their core while they're driving, waiting in line or brushing their teeth.

In addition to doing the exercises listed here, remember to do the **flexibility exercises** (pages 71–87) that target your problem areas.

specialty programs

CORE STRENGTH		
	64	lat release
	66	IT band release
	86	shoulder circles
	85	"hippest" hip stretch
	96	the hundred
	97	single-leg stretch
	98	rolling like a ball
	99	spine stretch forward
	103	ab lift
	104	ab lift with leg extension
	88	serratus anterior plank (modified to begin)

specialty programs
rotation

Increased rotation equals increased power, but all too often, the core muscles are weak and the spine isn't protected, therefore inciting injury to the back or spine. The most common complaint I receive from golfers is lower back injury and golf-related lower back pain. When the spine is supported in its natural curves, rotation is increased and the compression on the fragile discs between your vertebrae is decreased. *That* is healthy golf.

The key to rotation in golf is restoring full range of motion to your joints, especially your hips, shoulders and spine. Engaging in core work allows you to gain fuller rotation while protecting your back and spine from the shearing force that is generated from a powerful swing. With core work, you'll gain the knowledge and experience to keep your spine healthy and happy both during and after play.

In addition to doing the exercises listed here, remember to perform the **breathing exercises** (pages 58–60) as well as the **flexibility exercises** (pages 71–87) that target your trouble spots.

specialty programs

ROTATION		
	65	soften the buns
	66	IT band release
	67	inner thigh release
	70	lower back release
	81	rest pose
	84	knee over
	85	"hippest" hip stretch
	100	spine twist
	101	saw
	102	pendulum
	107	mermaid
	108	leg circles
	109	corkscrew
	117	single-leg twist

specialty programs
shoulder turn

Your shoulders connect your powerhouse and the club. If the connection is weak or limited, power won't be transferred efficiently. Flying elbows, lifting the head or shoulders and overswinging are a few swing faults that can occur when the shoulder joint is not moving with full range of motion and integrity.

Imagine your arms are like a light bulb that is plugging into its power source, your core, through your shoulder. If the connection is poor, the light bulb will flicker. If the light bulb is connected properly, the power surges through it and the bulb is illuminated with power.

As you study the musculature of the shoulder joint, focus on which muscles tend to be tight. Tight muscles lift the shoulders up around the ears and roll them forward, changing your center of gravity and causing upper-body dominance in golf. When your shoulders are down and wide, like a football player's, you are in a more powerful position for play.

Chances are, when you get to the end of your range of motion

SHOULDER TURN		
	61	neck release
	62	spine release
	63	back extension
	64	lat release
	69	chest release
	71	side and forward neck stretch
	72	neck turn
	76	shoulder and chest stretches
	78	crescent moon
	86	shoulder circles
	87	external shoulder rotation
	88	serratus anterior plank (modified to begin)
	91	draw a sword (standing)

with your backswing, you will still have some rotation left in your torso. Many golfers try to get a fuller backswing by letting their shoulders lift up and out of their core. Instead, rather than lifting the shoulders, take the shoulder turn to its end range and then see if you can rotate the torso.

specialty programs
hip turn

Much of the power in your swing comes from your ability to use your legs and feet against the ground. When your legs and feet are strong and supple, you'll be able to call upon the power they inherently possess. With full hip rotation, that power is transferred to and from the core easily. This program will give you a strong stance as well as fluid and even weight shift, and will help you keep your lower body connected to and working through your core.

Common imbalances in the hips and legs result in loss of spine angle, standing up or sitting down in the swing, hip sway and the reverse pivot. Limited range of motion in the hip area can cause stress to the area above the hip, generally the lower back, and at the knee. It's common for seniors to regain lost distance (15 to 25 yards in their drive) when range of motion is restored to the hips and legs.

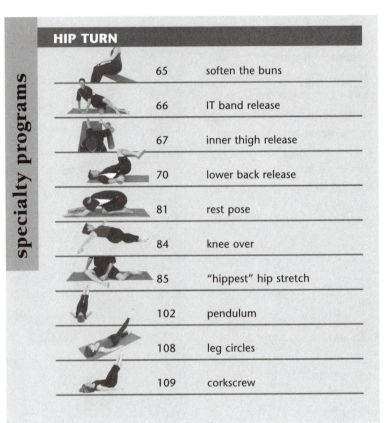

specialty programs

HIP TURN

	65	soften the buns
	66	IT band release
	67	inner thigh release
	70	lower back release
	81	rest pose
	84	knee over
	85	"hippest" hip stretch
	102	pendulum
	108	leg circles
	109	corkscrew

specialty programs
weight shift

During the full swing, 70 to 90 percent of your weight should shift onto your back leg and then to your follow-through leg. When I initially ask my golfer clients to balance on one leg, they're surprised to find it very challenging. Weight shift can be dramatically improved by balancing the entire system, especially the hips and legs, and by training with one-legged exercises.

Imbalances in the hip joint and injury of or surgery in the hips, knees and ankles can affect your ability to shift your weight in a fluid manner. The reverse pivot is a result of failing to shift the weight onto the front leg. The hip sway occurs when your hip stabilizers are weak; when you shift your weight, the hip continues to move beyond the standing foot, kind of like bumping the car door closed. For balance purposes, it should stop before it does the "bump" motion, and end up poised just above your standing foot.

specialty programs

WEIGHT SHIFT

	66	IT band release
	67	inner thigh release
	68	calf release
	85	"hippest" hip stretch
	84	knee over
	111	up and down
	113	standing balance
	114	weight shift
	115	standing leg circles
	112	split squat

part three:
the exercises

breathing
360-degree breath

As you practice the Pilates breathing during your workouts, your lunging pattern to emerge. This exercise uses an elastic band to give you feedback.

STARTING POSITION: Tie an elastic exercise band around your ribcage. It should feel firm, but not tight. Lie on your back in neutral spine angle with your knees bent and feet hip-width apart. Place your palms on the mat. **INHALE** through your nose. Relax your jaws and allow an audible **EXHALE** through your relaxed jaw. Avoid pursing your lips (as if blowing out a candle). Breathe in this manner, inhaling and exhaling 10 times to establish your natural breathing rhythm.

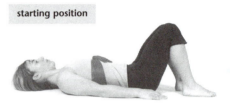

starting position

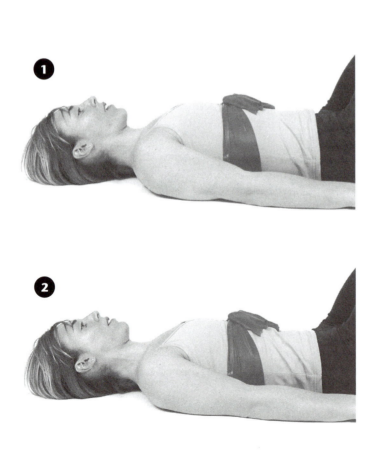

1 Once you have established a natural rhythm of breath, **INHALE**—expand your breath into the exercise band as if you're trying to stretch your ribcage into it in the front and the sides of your body. Feel your back expand toward the floor.

2 As you **EXHALE**, allow your ribs to relax naturally away from the band. Once you feel you have an understanding of the proper breathing pattern, practice by counting 10 cycles of breath.

GOLF BENEFITS
- Enhances the mind-body connection.
- Assists in relaxation and fluid tempo.

The standing version of the 360-degree breath challenges you to be aware of your sides and back while in neutral spine angle.

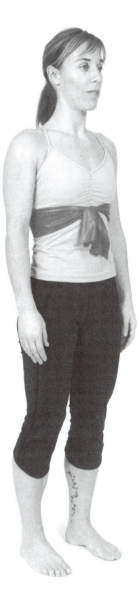

1 Stand in neutral spine angle with the band secured around your ribcage. **INHALE**, expanding the ribcage 360 degrees, into the front, sides and back of the body. **EXHALE**, allowing your ribs to relax away from the band. Once you have established the correct breathing pattern, count 10 cycles of breath.

GOLF BENEFITS

- Enhances the mind-body connection.
- Assists in relaxation and fluid tempo.

If you have a stability ball, you can use it to practice your breathing exercises. The goal is to learn to breathe into the sides and back of the body and overcome the tendency toward shallow chest breathing.

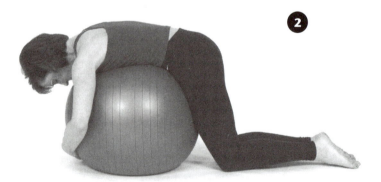

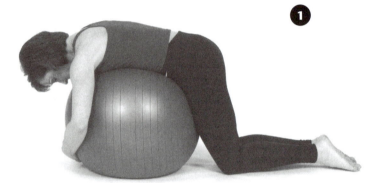

1 Lie on your belly over the ball as if you are draping yourself over it. **INHALE** through your nose, bringing your breath into the rib area on the sides and back of your body.

2 **EXHALE**, softening your ribs away from the skin.

GOLF BENEFITS

- Expands your lungs more fully, enhancing your ability to bring blood and oxygen to your system
- Increases upper torso flexibility for greater rotation through your swing.
- Assists in relaxation during movement.

neck release   *target: neck*

Caution: Neck exercises should be done with the utmost care as the neck can be fragile. Think of "good hurt, bad hurt." If you experience "bad hurt" during neck exercises, stop and consult a professional.

STARTING POSITION: Lie on your back with your knees bent and your feet flat on the floor. Align your heels with your buttocks and make sure you have equal weight across the balls of your feet. Place the roller behind your neck, resting your neck and the base of your skull on it. **INHALE** to begin.

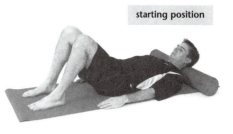

starting position

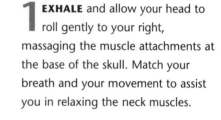

1 EXHALE and allow your head to roll gently to your right, massaging the muscle attachments at the base of the skull. Match your breath and your movement to assist you in relaxing the neck muscles.

2 INHALE back to center, then **EXHALE** and repeat to the left.

Continue breathing and massaging your neck for 2 to 3 minutes or until it feels relaxed and released.

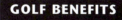

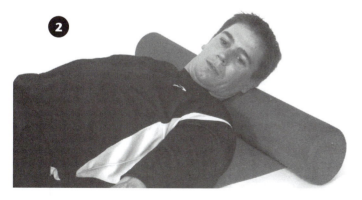

GOLF BENEFITS

• Releases neck and shoulder tension while increasing mobility and range of motion.
• Increases shoulder turn and ability to keep head in the proper position and eyes on the ball.

STARTING POSITION: Lie on your back with your knees bent and hips, knees and toes aligned. Keep equal weight on the balls of your feet. Place the roller behind your back at the lower edge of your shoulder blades. Place your hands behind your head; keep your elbows in your peripheral vision. Relax your chin toward your chest and focus your eyes on your knees or belly. **INHALE** to begin.

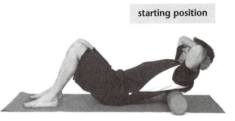

starting position

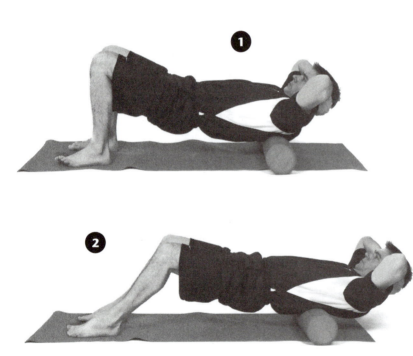

1 **EXHALE** and lift your hips toward the ceiling. Breathing continuously, roll the roller up and down your spine, to the top of your shoulder blades and to the bottom of the ribcage area. Don't roll onto the lower lumbar area.

2 When you find tight or tender areas, stop, breathe and sink your body weight into the area, allowing it to relax into the roller.

Roll up and down until your spine is fully released.

GOLF BENEFITS

• Releases tight muscles and connective tissue in the mid to upper area of the spine, increasing range of motion for greater torso turn.

back extension

target: spine

Back extension may feel uncomfortable at first, but stay with it. If you have a spinal condition, however, consult with your physician prior to doing this exercise.

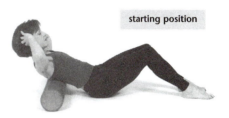

starting position

STARTING POSITION: Lie on your back with your knees bent and hips, knees and toes aligned; keep equal weight on the balls of your feet. Place the roller behind your back at the lower edge of your shoulder blades. Place your hands behind your head, keeping your elbows in your peripheral vision.

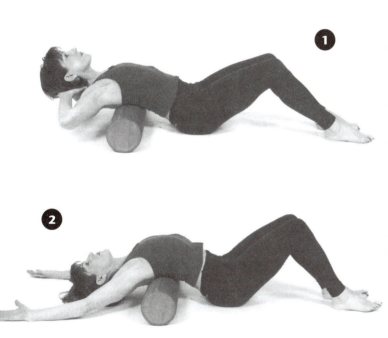

1 Keeping your hips on the floor, **INHALE** and open your chest toward the ceiling, increasing the space between your pelvis and your chest. Allow your upper body to drape over the roller, curving your spine backward. **EXHALE**, relaxing into this back bend.

2 When you begin to feel comfortable in the back extension, release your neck and drape your arms over the top of the roller, resting your head on the floor.

GOLF BENEFITS

- Increases range of motion in the spine for enhanced swing play.
- Releases the tight muscles of the chest, the front of the shoulders and neck.

STARTING POSITION: Lie on your back with the roller beneath your shoulder blades. Roll onto your right side, draping your right arm over the roller. Make a fist with your right hand and point your thumb as if you were hitchhiking; turn your thumb toward the ceiling. Lean your weight forward so that your right hip is directly over your left hip. The roller should end up in the lower edge of your armpit at the attachment of your lat muscle. If you have tightness in your lat, you will feel discomfort when you roll onto it.

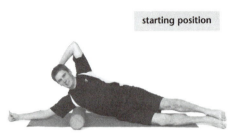

starting position

1 Once you find the lat, sink your weight into it and breathe continuously, giving it 45 seconds to 1 minute to release. The discomfort should decrease substantially once it releases.

Upon release, roll onto your back then to your left side, repeating the release.

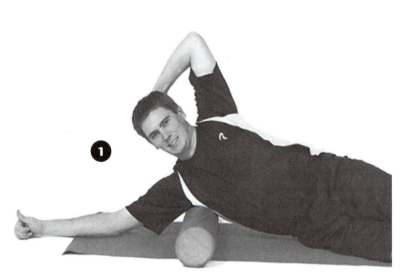

GOLF BENEFITS

• Generates more power by increasing your ability to turn.
• Increases accuracy by allowing you to stay on your swing plane.

STARTING POSITION: Sit on the roller with your knees bent and feet flat in front of you.

starting position

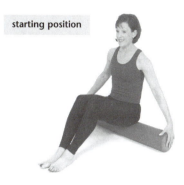

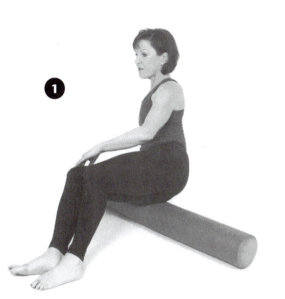

1 Lean your weight onto your right buttock, placing your right hand on the floor behind the roller. As you roll on your buttock, feel for any tight or tender areas. Relax your weight into those areas while breathing continuously for 45 seconds to 1 minute.

Return to center and repeat on your left side.

MODIFICATION

If you have the flexibility, place the ankle of the buttock you're releasing onto your left knee.

GOLF BENEFITS

• Increases hip turn and reduces lower back pain by releasing the piriformis muscles in your buttocks.

roller release
IT band release

The iliotibial (IT) band, a wide swath of connective tissue on the outer leg from hip to knee, is often tight and especially tender. It may take a few weeks to work through the discomfort.

STARTING POSITION: Sit on the roller with your legs extended in front of you. Keeping your right leg extended, roll the roller under the outside of your right thigh, just below your hip joint. Place your hands on the floor behind the roller. Bend your left leg, crossing it in front of your right, and place your left foot on the floor.

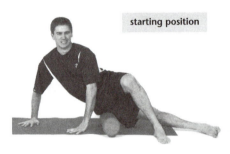

starting position

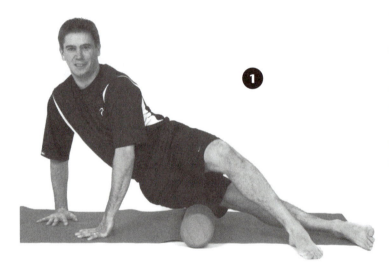

1 Breathing continuously, slowly roll down your IT band toward your knee. Stop in any tight or tender areas, giving them 45 seconds to 1 minute to release. Stop just above your knee joint.

Return to center and repeat on your left side.

GOLF BENEFITS

• Increases hip turn and enhances fluid weight shift.

inner thigh release   *target: thigh*

Another tender area, but worth the discomfort!

STARTING POSITION: Lie on your belly with the roller on your left side parallel to your body. Bend your left knee and place the roller under your lower leg from your knee to your ankle. Place your forearms flat on the floor in front of you. Pull your shoulders away from your ears. Lift your belly toward the ceiling to support your lower back.

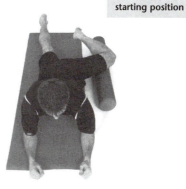

starting position

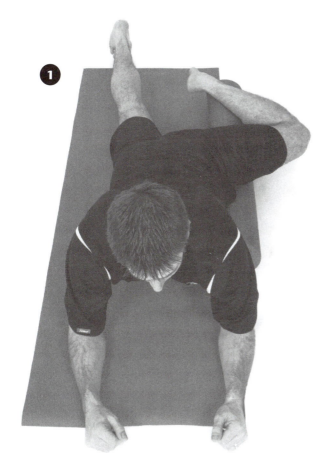

1 Breathe continuously as you roll on your inner thigh toward your groin and back toward your knee, but don't roll onto your knee joint.

Allow any areas of tightness or tenderness 45 seconds to 1 minute to release.

GOLF BENEFITS

• Enhances hip turn and strength in the stance.

roller release
calf release
target: calf

STARTING POSITION: Sit on the floor with your legs extended in front of you, your calves resting on the roller. **INHALE** to begin.

starting position

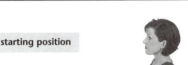

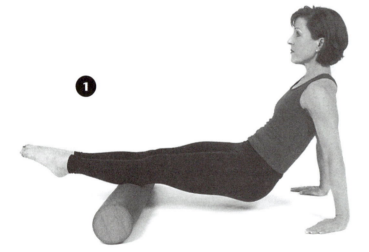

1 EXHALE, pressing your hands into the floor to lift your hips away from the floor and shift your weight onto your calves. Keep your shoulders down and away from your ears. Breathing continuously, roll the roller up and down your calves by bending and straightening your knees, stopping in any tight or tender areas to allow them time to release. Try also rocking your calves from side to side on the roller. Be careful not to apply pressure behind the knee.

GOLF BENEFITS

- Reduces ankle, knee and foot problems, contributing to a strong stance and weight shift.

chest release   *target: chest, front shoulder*

STARTING POSITION: Lie with your spine on the roller, making sure your head and buttocks are supported. Bend your knees and place your feet hip-width apart on the floor, aligning your hips, knees and toes. Place equal weight across the balls of your feet. Keep your chest relaxed and your back ribs connected to the roller. Maintain neutral spine angle throughout the movement. Lift your arms up to the ceiling and press your palms together, then bend your elbows to a right angle, allowing your forearms to meet and your hands to point over your head. Keep your elbows over your shoulders and your elbows and wrists at the same height.

starting position

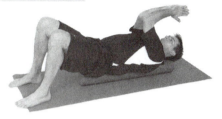

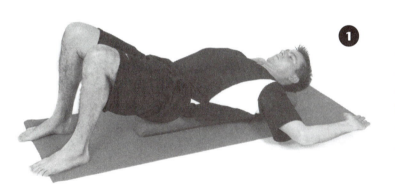

1 INHALE and then **EXHALE.** Keeping your arms bent at a right angle, allow them to part in opposite directions. They will naturally stop at the end of their flexibility. Relax in this position, breathing continuously for at least 1 minute. Most people relax up to 5 minutes in this stretch.

MODIFICATION

Use a small pillow to support your arm if needed.

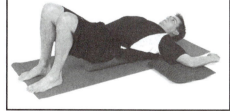

GOLF BENEFITS

- Increases the range of motion at the shoulder joint for maximum swing arc, helping you stay on your swing plane and increasing power through your downswing.

A great post-game stretch to prevent lower back soreness.

STARTING POSITION: Place the roller under your lower back so it cradles and supports your lumbar spine. Keep the roller in the lumbar curve or a bit lower to support the spine and pelvis. Don't arch the spine and the front ribs toward the ceiling. Drop your shoulders away from your ears. Immediately lift your knees toward the ceiling.

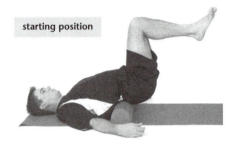

starting position

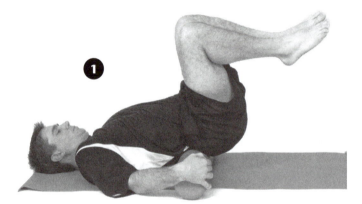

①

1–2 Breathing continuously, move your knees from side to side, massaging the area around the sacrum, the bony triangle at the base of your spine. Hold the ends of the roller for support if necessary.

Spend 1–3 minutes releasing.

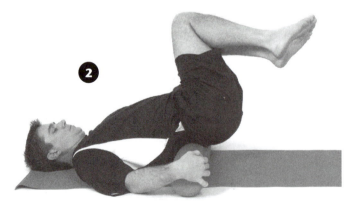

②

GOLF BENEFITS

• Releases lower back, increasing range of motion for greater hip turn.

side and forward neck stretch | *target: neck*

Focus on your breath to assist in releasing tight or tense areas.

STARTING POSITION: Stand in address stance with neutral spine angle. **INHALE** to begin.

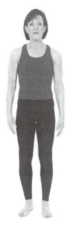

starting position

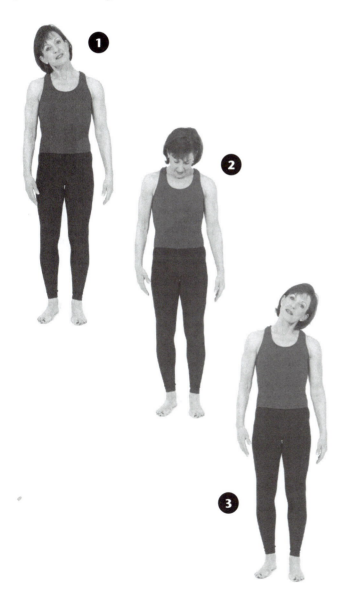

1 **EXHALE** while slowly drawing your right ear toward your right shoulder.

2 **INHALE** and then **EXHALE** while gently rolling your head forward, placing your chin toward your chest. Don't roll your head around with momentum.

3 **INHALE** and then **EXHALE** while gently rolling your head to the left, as if you're going to place your left ear on your left shoulder.

INHALE and **EXHALE** to return to center and repeat to the left. Roll slowly side to side 5 times.

GOLF BENEFITS
- Increases range of motion in the neck and shoulders for greater shoulder turn.
- Helps you keep your eyes on the ball.

neck turn

target: neck

STARTING POSITION: Stand in address stance in neutral spine angle. **INHALE** to begin.

starting position

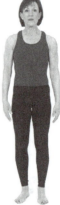

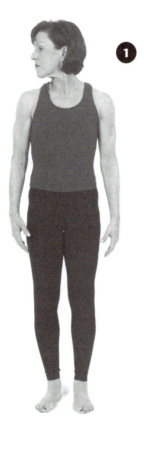

1

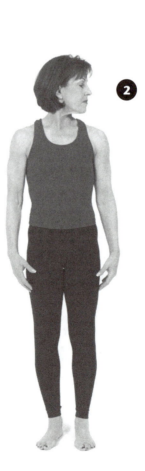

2

1 **EXHALE** while turning your head to the right, as if to look over your right shoulder. Keep your nose in alignment with your chin and your eyes level with the horizon; don't tilt your head. Breathe continuously while gently holding this twisting stretch for 45 seconds.

2 **INHALE** to return to center and **EXHALE** to repeat to the left side.

GOLF BENEFITS

• Increases neck flexibility in rotation, allowing your head to remain forward, eyes looking at the ball, while your shoulders turn in full swing.

This is a great stretch to do in between shots if you tend to give the club the death grip.

STARTING POSITION: Stand in address stance with neutral spine angle. Begin with your hands relaxed in front of you. **INHALE** to begin.

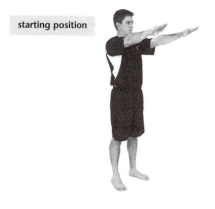

starting position

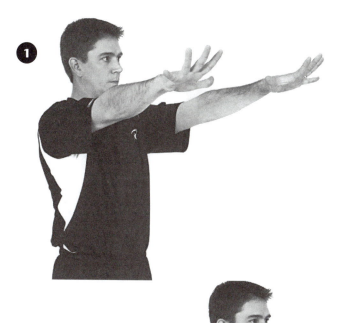

1 EXHALE while stretching the hands open; spread your fingers as wide as possible.

2 INHALE to relax your hands.

Repeat 10 times.

GOLF BENEFITS

• Keeps the hands supple for a relaxed grip.

STARTING POSITION: Stand in address stance with neutral spine angle. Extend both arms in front of you to shoulder height. Place your palms together in opposite directions so that your fingertips reach just to the fold of the opposite wrist. **INHALE** to begin.

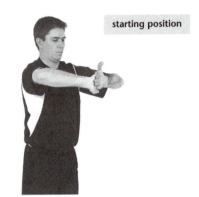

starting position

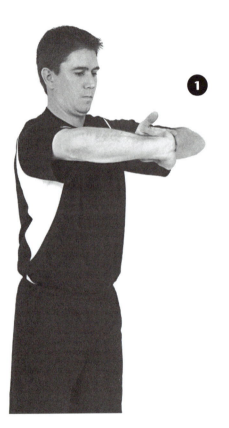

1

1 EXHALE while gently pressing your palms toward one another for a count of 10. **INHALE** to release.

Repeat 10 times. Change hand positions.

GOLF BENEFITS

- Balances flexibility in the forearm for more precise wrist cock.
- Releases the hands for a relaxed grip.

STARTING POSITION: Stand in address stance with neutral spine angle. Extend your right arm forward and fold your wrist so that your palm faces toward your body and your fingers point toward the floor in a stretch. **INHALE** to begin.

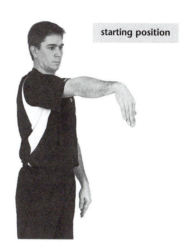

starting position

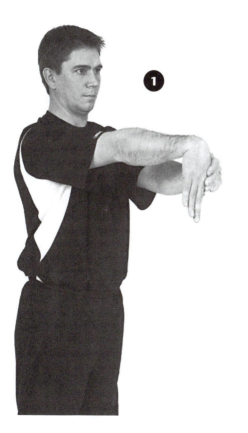

1 Place your left palm on your right hand. **EXHALE** while applying pressure with your left hand, increasing the depth of the stretch slowly, counting to 10. **INHALE** to release.

Repeat 10 times. Change hands.

GOLF BENEFITS

- Increases wrist flexibility for better position when cocking the wrists.
- Helps to keep the hands relaxed for better wrist release.

Tightness in the chest and shoulders may cause your shoulders to rise up around your ears in these exercises. Keep your shoulders back and down throughout these stretches. You may not get your elbows straight, but that will come in time.

STARTING POSITION: Stand in address stance with neutral spine angle.

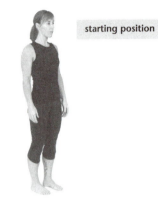

starting position

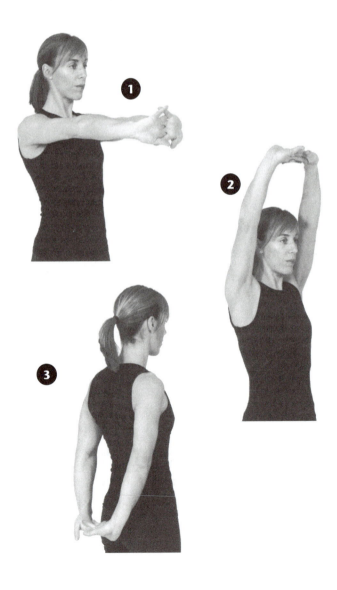

STRETCH 1 Inhale while extending your arms in front of you, lacing your fingers. Exhale and face your palms away from you. Try to straighten your elbows so they are fully extended but not locked. Imagine you are pressing your palms against a wall. Breathe continuously. Hold for 45 seconds.

STRETCH 2 From Stretch 1, raise your arms above your head. Imagine you are pressing your palms against the ceiling. Breathe continuously. Hold for 45 seconds.

STRETCH 3 From Starting Position, inhale while extending your arms behind your back and lacing your fingers. (Hold a golf towel between your hands if they do not reach one another comfortably.) Exhale and stretch your arms back and up as if you're going to slide them up a wall behind you. Don't let your chest and ribs splay forward.

If you experience shoulder pain after making modifications, stop and consult with a professional before continuing shoulder exercises.

STARTING POSITION: Lie on your right side with your knees bent, shoulders and hips stacked atop one another. Cradle your head on your right arm. Extend your left arm in front of you so that it's straight but not locked.

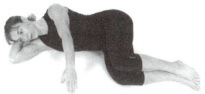

starting position

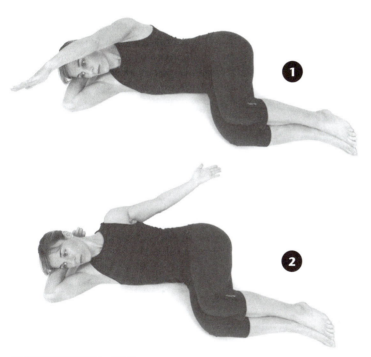

1

2

1 **INHALE** while slowly and carefully sweeping your left arm overhead and back behind you. Imagine you have a paintbrush in your hand and are painting a circle.

2 **EXHALE** as you continue making the circle, sweeping your arm down toward your toes, returning to starting position.

Circle 8 times, then circle 8 times in the opposite direction. Change sides and repeat with the right arm.

MODIFICATION

If you have shoulder issues, bend your elbow and make smaller circles.

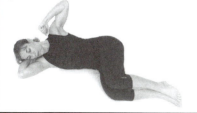

GOLF BENEFITS

• Increases range of motion of the shoulder joints for maximum backswing and follow-through.

STARTING POSITION: Stand in address stance in neutral spine angle. Inhale to extend your arms overhead and press your palms together. While exhaling, draw your shoulders away from your ears and lift your ribcage away from your pelvis. Imagine your waistline is like a tube of toothpaste, squeezed in the center and elongating at the ends. Keep your head and shoulders in line with your hips throughout the movement. **INHALE** and try to reach the ceiling with your hands.

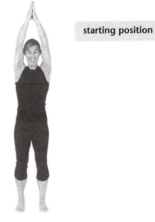

starting position

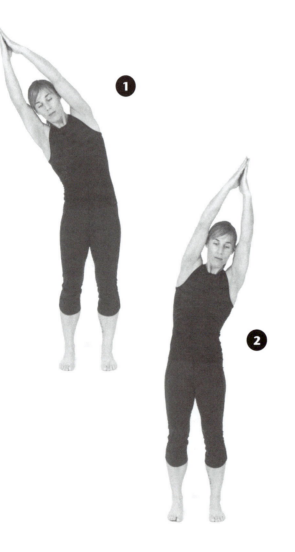

❶

❷

1 **EXHALE** and bend from your waist to the right. Don't twist or rotate your upper body to try to stretch further. Breathe continuously, holding the stretch for 45 seconds.

2 **INHALE** back to center and then **EXHALE**, stretching from your waist to the left.

GOLF BENEFITS

• Enhances hip turn in both directions.

STARTING POSITION: Stand in address stance with neutral spine angle. Imagine there's a wall behind you.

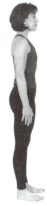

starting position

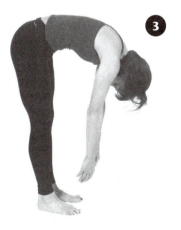

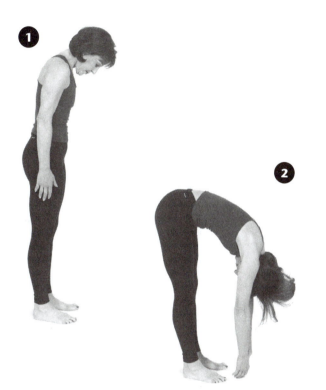

1 Breathe continuously as you slowly peel your spine off the wall one vertebra at a time, beginning with your chin to your chest. Imagine rolling the top of your head into your belly to activate the stretch.

2 Continue peeling with your chest to your ribs and your ribs to your pelvis until you are in a forward bend. Bend your knees if you need to. Look at your navel or between your legs to release your neck.

3 Return to your upright stance, placing one vertebra at a time back on the wall. Your neck and head should come up last.

GOLF BENEFITS

- Hamstring flexibility makes holding the proper spine angle easier.
- Spinal flexibility increases turning potential for a bigger swing.

target: spine

STARTING POSITION: Begin in Belly-Down position, legs straight and together. Keep your feet on the floor throughout the movement. Place your arms on the floor at a 90-degree bend with your elbows in line with your shoulders. Keep your shoulders away from your ears and draw your navel to your spine to support your lower back. **INHALE** to begin.

starting position

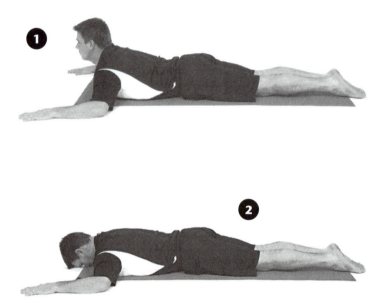

1—2 **EXHALE** while lengthening your upper body forward and then up, as if you were rolling a marble to the wall in front of you with your nose. Lift one vertebra at a time toward the ceiling, keeping your neck aligned with the rest of your spine. **INHALE** at the top of the movement, then **EXHALE** while releasing one vertebra at a time to the floor.

Repeat 8 times.

GOLF BENEFITS

- Decreases potential for lower back pain.
- Strengthens neutral spine angle.
- Trains proper positioning of shoulders for greatest power transfer from core to club.

Use this stretch anytime you need to regroup and re-energize. If this bothers your knees and/or ankles, place a rolled-up towel behind your knees and/or under your ankles.

STARTING POSITION: Begin in Hands and Knees position.

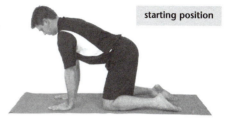

starting position

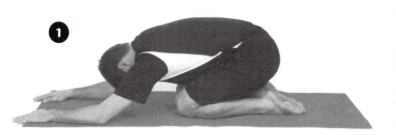

1 Shift your buttocks back to sit on your heels. Extend your arms and hands over your head, keeping them in line with your shoulders; keep your shoulders away from your ears. If possible, rest your buttocks on your heels and your head on the floor. Breathe continuously, resting for 45 seconds to 1 minute.

GOLF BENEFITS

• Allows your mind and body to integrate the movement exercises you have been working with.

lat stretch

target: lats

This variation on Draw a Sword (page 90) is a favorite of my golfers.

STARTING POSITION: Begin on your knees and elbows. Keep your knees directly under your hips and your elbows under your shoulders.

starting position

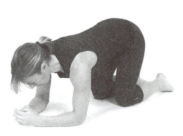

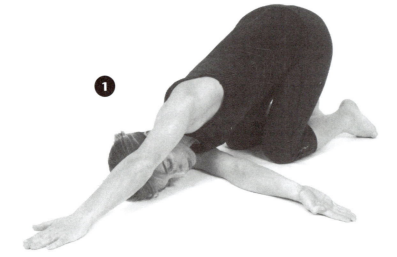

1 **INHALE** and reach your right arm through the space between your left arm and left knee. **EXHALE**, actively stretching your right side from your back through your fingertips as you continue to reach to your left side. Keep your shoulders away from your ears and keep your knees under your hips. Shift your weight to your right side to intensify the stretch; don't let your hips drop toward your heels. Rest your head on the floor. Hold for 45 seconds to 1 minute.

Repeat on the left side.

GOLF BENEFITS

• Increases shoulder and torso turn for maximum swing arc.

This is a preparation for the Split Squat exercise (page 112).

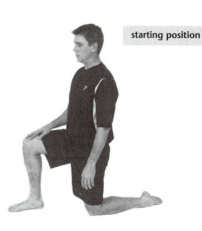

starting position

STARTING POSITION: Begin in a kneeling lunge with your left knee on the floor and your right knee in front of your right hip, the right ankle directly under the knee. Your left knee should be directly under your left hip, with your left foot lined up behind your knee. Stay in neutral spine angle while activating the stretch.

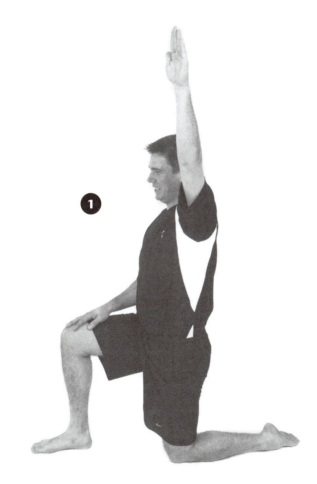

1 Place your right hand on your right knee. Raise your left hand over your head, lengthening your left side from hip to fingertips. Breathing continuously, draw your navel to your spine and lengthen your lower back. Don't allow your tailbone to stick out behind you like a duck's behind. Hold for 45 seconds.

Change legs and repeat on the other side.

GOLF BENEFITS

- Increases flexibility in the stance muscles for a stronger stance.
- Prevents lower back tightness for greater hip turn.

knee over   *target: shoulders, chest, hips, sides of body*

STARTING POSITION: Lie on your back with your knees bent and feet flat on the floor. Stretch your arms out to the sides into a "T."

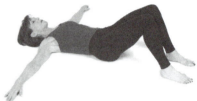

starting position

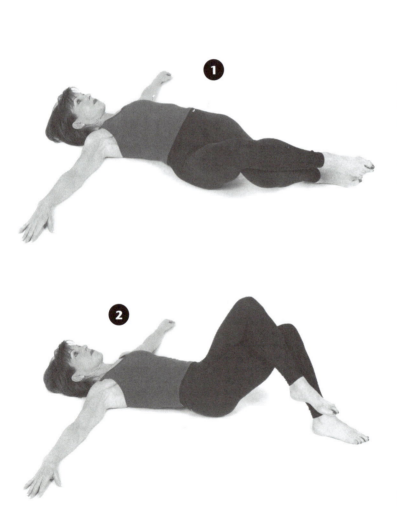

1 Cross your right knee over your left knee and then **INHALE**. **EXHALE** while smoothly lowering both knees to your right side, twisting at your waistline. Don't let your ribcage splay toward the ceiling as you twist; keep your ribcage relaxed.

2 **INHALE** and then **EXHALE** to press your lower back to the floor and draw your navel to your spine, using your abdominal muscles to return your knees to center. Cross your left leg over your right and repeat.

Do 10 side-to-side movements.

GOLF BENEFITS
• Increases hip and torso flexibility for increased power.

"hippest" hip stretch
target: hips

Avoid this exercise if you've had a serious knee injury. If your hips are very inflexible, place a small pillow or rolled-up towel under the hip of the forward leg.

STARTING POSITION: Begin seated in neutral spine with your knees bent in front of you.

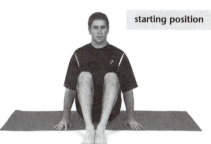

starting position

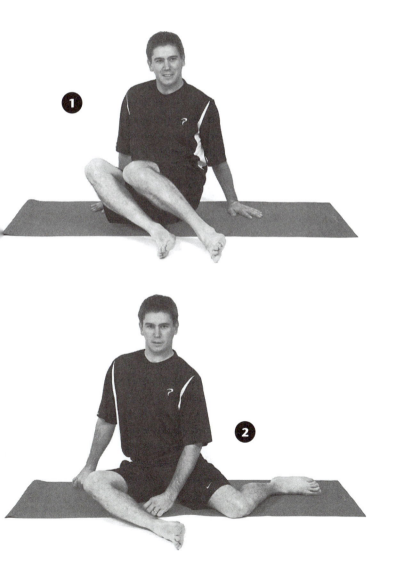

1 Fold both knees to the right and align your hips so that they both point forward. Line up your right thigh bone so that it points straight ahead and your lower leg is at a 90-degree angle to the left.

2 Now align your left leg by sliding it to the left, trying to get your left thigh bone to point directly to your left with the lower leg at a 90-degree angle. Place your right hand on the floor close to your right hip for support. Breathe continuously, relaxing your left hip toward the floor. Your goal is to gain enough flexibility to place both hips evenly on the floor and facing straight ahead of you. Hold this position for 45-60 seconds.

Change sides and repeat.

GOLF BENEFITS
- Opens the hips for increased rotation.
- Helps reduce lower back pain.

target: chest, shoulders

For this exercise, notice how your arms are connected to your core and try to initiate all movement from your core rather than your hands. Imagine you have balloons tied to your wrists.

STARTING POSITION: Lie on your back in neutral spine angle with your knees bent and your feet flat on the floor; keep your knees aligned with your hips. Place your arms by your sides with your palms down. Keep your shoulders away from your ears throughout the exercise.

starting position

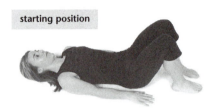

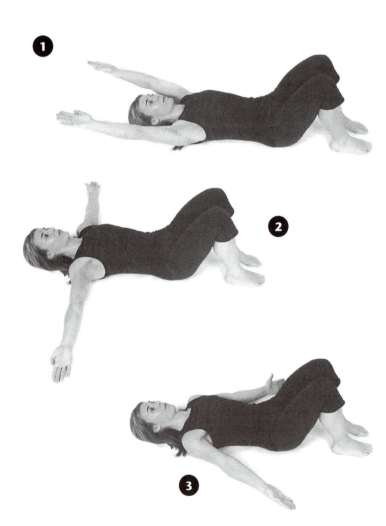

1 **INHALE** and allow your hands to float to the ceiling and then over your head. Don't let your back ribs lift away from the floor.

2 **EXHALE** and circle your arms down as if making the letter "T" with your upper body.

3 Slide your shoulder blades down your back to return your arms to your sides.

Draw 10 slow circles, then repeat in the opposite direction.

GOLF BENEFITS

• Increases the connection of the golf club to the core.
• Decreases the tendency to overuse the arms through the swing.

external shoulder rotation
target: shoulders

It's sometimes helpful to hold a small towel between your elbow and your side to maintain the proper position.

STARTING POSITION: Lie on your right side with knees bent; cradle your head with your right arm. Place your left elbow at your waist. Make a fist and bend your elbow 90 degrees; your forearm and hand will be at waist height. **INHALE** to begin.

starting position

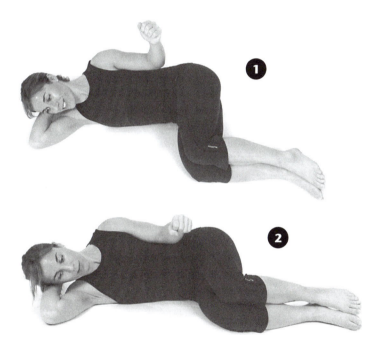

1 Keeping your elbow attached to your side, **EXHALE** while lifting your fist toward the ceiling. Make sure your wrist doesn't bend.

2 **INHALE** and slowly return to starting position.

Do 10 movements and repeat on the other side.

ADVANCED

Try this by sitting in a chair (or on the floor) in neutral spine angle and holding an elastic exercise band in both hands, anchoring your elbows to your sides.

GOLF BENEFITS

- This protects one of the rotator cuff muscles that is prone to golf injury.
- Trains correct elbow position in backswing and follow-through.

STARTING POSITION: Lie in Belly-Down position. Place your elbows on the floor directly under your shoulders with your forearms and fingers facing forward. **INHALE** to begin.

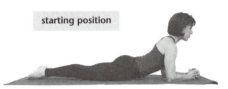

starting position

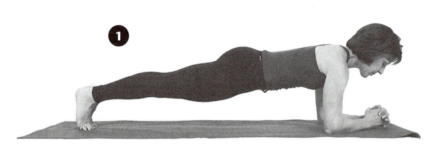

1 **EXHALE** and lift your torso and knees off the floor while maintaining neutral spine. Activate the connection between your navel and your spine to support your lower back; don't let your belly sag. Keep your head aligned with your neck, which should, in turn, be aligned with the rest of the spine. Hold the plank for 20 seconds.

Release the knees to the floor to rest, then repeat 3 to 6 times.

MODIFICATION

Keep your knees on the floor as you lift your torso so that you are supporting your weight on your forearms and knees.

GOLF BENEFITS

• Increases the power transfer from the core to the club.

serratus anterior push-ups
target: shoulders, back

This is an advanced version of the Serratus Anterior Plank (page 88).

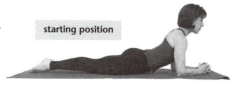

starting position

STARTING POSITION: Lie in Belly-Down position. Place your elbows on the floor directly under your shoulders with your forearms and fingers facing forward. **INHALE** to begin.

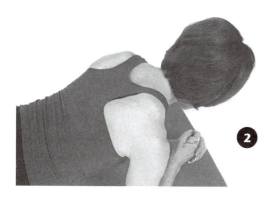

1 **EXHALE** and lift your torso and knees off the floor while maintaining neutral spine. Activate the connection between your navel and your spine to support your lower back; don't let your belly sag. Keep your head aligned with your neck, which should, in turn, be aligned with the rest of the spine.

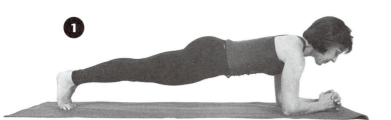

2 **INHALE**, lowering your torso toward the floor the floor, keeping your spine in a neutral position. Your shoulder blades will slide in and up.

3 **EXHALE** and lift your torso back up to step 1.

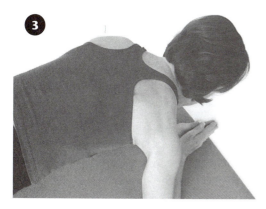

Repeat 6 times to begin, working up to 10 times. Release your knees to the floor to rest.

GOLF BENEFITS

- Increases the power transfer from the core to the club.

target: back, chest, shoulders

As you move through each segment of the exercise, think shoulder-elbow-hand, and then hand-elbow-shoulder to return.

STARTING POSITION: Begin on your knees and elbows, with your knees directly under your hips and your elbows under your shoulders, forearms facing forward. Keep your shoulders away from your ears throughout the movement.

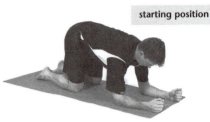

starting position

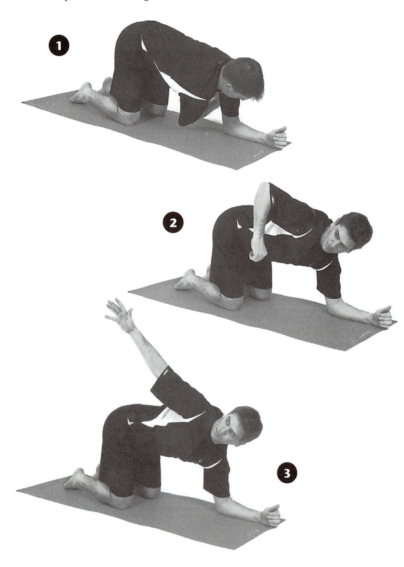

1 INHALE and reach your right arm through the space between your left elbow and left knee. Initiate the movement from your core rather than from your arm or hand. **EXHALE** and actively stretch your right side from your back through your fingertips.

2 INHALE and draw your right shoulder blade toward your spine and your elbow to the ceiling.

3 EXHALE and extend your arm, rotate your chest toward the ceiling and look up at your fingertips. **INHALE** to reverse the motion back to step 1.

Repeat 10 times and switch sides.

GOLF BENEFITS

• Trains the muscle movement and firing pattern for the backswing and follow-through.

draw a sword (standing) *target: core, back shoulder*

A slow and even return works your muscles in eccentric contraction. This is especially good protection for the shoulder. This is a more advanced version of Draw a Sword (page 90).

STARTING POSITION: Stand in address stance with an elastic exercise band anchored under your left foot. Hold the other end of the band in your right hand, close to your left thigh. **INHALE** to begin.

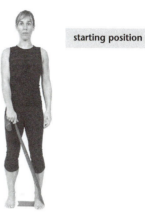

starting position

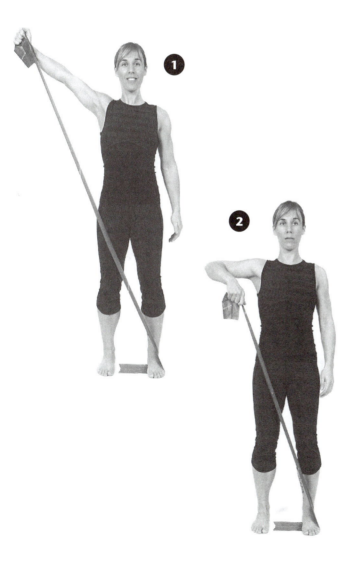

1 **EXHALE** while drawing your right shoulder blade toward your spine, your elbow out to your side and then extending your right arm fully as if you are drawing a sword.

2 **INHALE**, reversing the motion slowly as you return your sword to its scabbard and yourself to center.

Repeat 10 times and switch sides.

GOLF BENEFITS

- Strengthens the take-away and follow-through muscles.
- Trains core-to-club connection for greater power.

stability & strength series
side lift
target: shoulders, core

92

This exercise trains the integration of the shoulder girdle to the core.

STARTING POSITION: Lie on your left side with your left elbow directly under your shoulder. Extend your legs and scissor your right leg in front of your left, keeping both feet on the ground. Try to align your ear to shoulder to hip to ankle. Place your right hand on the floor in front of you. Keep your shoulders away from your ears and look straight ahead throughout the exercise. **INHALE** to begin.

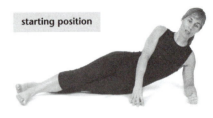

starting position

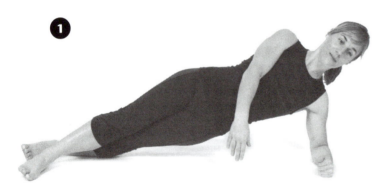

1

1 EXHALE as you activate your core muscles to lift your hips off the floor. Be careful to keep the bottom of your shoulder connected to your core. **INHALE** as you slowly return your hips to the floor.

Repeat 5 times, then switch sides. Eventually work up to 10 movements on each side.

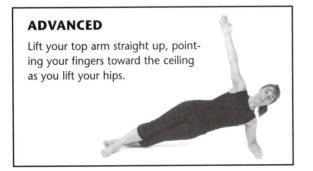

ADVANCED

Lift your top arm straight up, pointing your fingers toward the ceiling as you lift your hips.

GOLF BENEFITS

• Increases the transfer of power from the core to the club.

This is a great full-body strengthener. Caution: Plank in any position can stress the shoulder joint if not executed properly. Be certain you can keep your shoulders down and supported by your core before attempting a full plank.

starting position

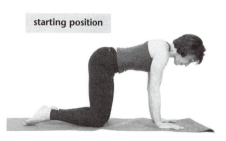

STARTING POSITION: Begin in Hands and Knees position, with your hands under your shoulders and your knees under your hips. Keep your head and neck aligned throughout the movement. **INHALE** to begin.

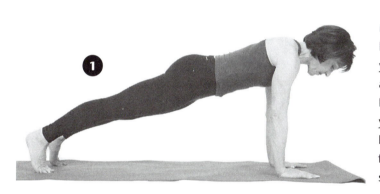

1 EXHALE and draw your navel to your spine while extending your right leg, then your left, straight behind you, forming a plank with your body. Imagine your spine is like a steel rod, strong and straight. Don't round your upper back or lift your buttocks into the air, and don't let your midsection sag toward the floor. Hold the position for 20 seconds, breathing continuously.

To release the movement, lower your knees and move into Rest Pose (page 81) for 20 seconds. Repeat 5 times.

GOLF BENEFITS

- A full-body strength exercise for increasing power from core to club.

94

This is a great full-body strengthener.

STARTING POSITION: Begin in Hands and Knees position. Extend your right leg directly behind you to touch the ball of your foot to the floor. Place your right hand on your hip while you pivot on your left knee and hand to face the right side. Align your right ear, shoulder, hip and ankle into a straight line. **INHALE** to begin.

starting position

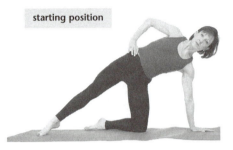

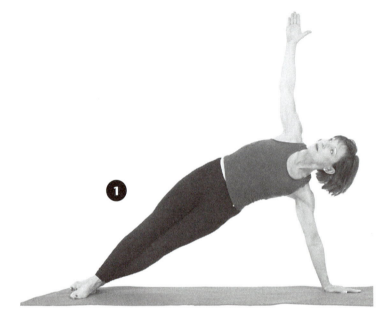

1 EXHALE while activating your core muscles, and slide your left leg out to place your left foot just behind your right foot. At the same time, extend your right arm to the ceiling so that your arms are stretching in opposite directions. Hold for 20 seconds, breathing continuously.

INHALE to return to starting position. Repeat 5 times and switch sides.

SUPER-ADVANCED

From full side plank position, inhale then exhale to activate your core. Lift your hips toward the ceiling and rotate your torso while sweeping your upper arm under your waist.

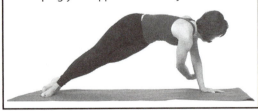

GOLF BENEFITS

- A full-body exercise to develop a more powerful swing.
- The advanced version enhances power from the core to the club through stronger rotation.

side arm pitch

target: obliques, core, spine

STARTING POSITION: Secure one end of an elastic exercise band to a stable object (such as a table or chair leg) at knee height or lower. Hold the other end in both hands. Position yourself so that the secured end of the band is on your left side. Stand with your feet a little wider than your address stance and in neutral spine angle. **INHALE** to begin.

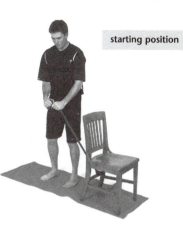

starting position

1 EXHALE while activating your core muscles to lift your arms and hands diagonally from your left leg to the height of your right shoulder. Don't let your hands get ahead of your torso.

2 INHALE while slowly reversing the movement.

GOLF BENEFITS

- Trains and strengthens the muscle-firing pattern of the backswing.
- Increases flexibility for the follow-through.

If your back hurts in this exercise, lift your legs more toward the ceiling until your abdominals get stronger. Or keep your legs on the ground instead of raising them.

STARTING POSITION: Lie in Knees to Ceiling position, with your arms and fingers off the floor, reaching for your toes. **INHALE** then **EXHALE** to the Peel-Up position while extending your legs toward the ceiling. Imagine gliding your ribcage toward your pelvis like folding the pleats of an accordion. Keep your lower back on the floor.

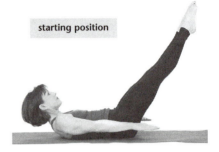

starting position

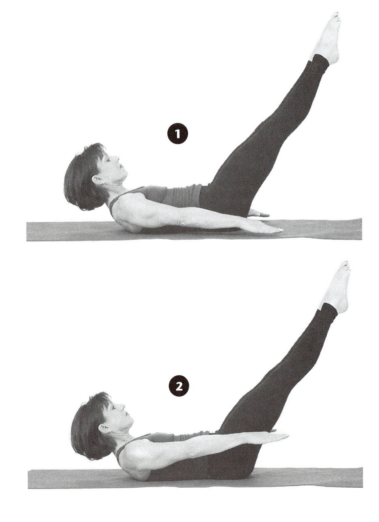

1 **INHALE** 4 short breaths, pumping your arms in small movements like you are slapping water.

2 **EXHALE** 6 short percussive breaths, coordinating the movement of your arms to the percussion of your breath. Continue to draw your navel to your spine with each exhale. Place your hand behind your head for support if your neck becomes fatigued.

Continue inhaling and exhaling with that pattern, counting in 10s until you reach 10 cycles, equaling 100 counts.

GOLF BENEFITS
- Elongates the spine for increased rotation through the golf swing.
- Teaches pelvic stability for reduced hip sway.

stability & strength series
single-leg stretch
target: core

97

STARTING POSITION: Begin in Knees to Ceiling position, then move into the Peel-Up position, keeping your neck long by looking at your navel. Extend your left leg to the ceiling while placing both hands on your right knee. Don't let your knees point out to the sides; instead, try to keep them aligned with your hips. Maintain neutral spine angle throughout the exercise, keeping your lower back connected to the floor. **INHALE** to begin.

starting position

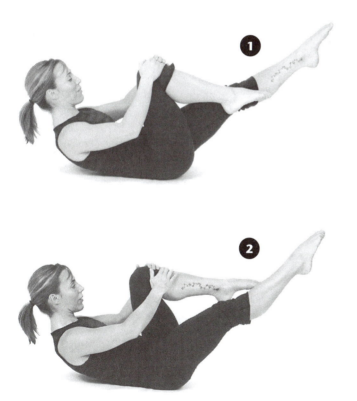

1 **EXHALE** while extending your left leg diagonally. Use your abdominal and pelvic-floor strength to keep your pelvis still while moving your legs. If your lower back arches away from the floor, you have gone too far.

2 **INHALE** to center, then **EXHALE** while changing legs and the position of your hands. Extend your right leg diagonally.

Continue the breathing pattern while changing legs 10 times.

GOLF BENEFITS
- Strengthens the core, quadriceps and hip flexors for a more stable stance.
- Increases flexibility in the hips for better hip turn.

Although this looks simple, it's not easy, especially for those with tight lower backs. If you can roll down but can't come back up, just roll onto your side and press up to the start position. As your back lengthens and your abdominals get stronger, rolling will get easier.

STARTING POSITION: Sit on your sitting bones with your knees bent close to your body, arms hugging your lower legs, toes just off the floor. Keep your heels as close to your body as possible.

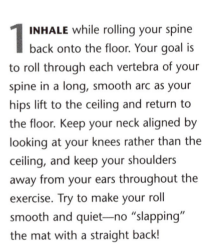

starting position

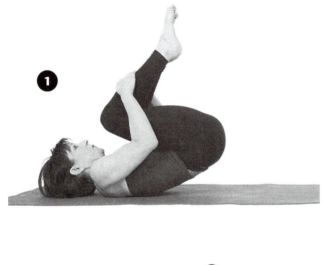

1 INHALE while rolling your spine back onto the floor. Your goal is to roll through each vertebra of your spine in a long, smooth arc as your hips lift to the ceiling and return to the floor. Keep your neck aligned by looking at your knees rather than the ceiling, and keep your shoulders away from your ears throughout the exercise. Try to make your roll smooth and quiet—no "slapping" the mat with a straight back!

2 EXHALE while rolling your spine forward and your hips toward the floor, stopping before your toes touch the floor. Don't throw your head and shoulders forward in an attempt to come back up.

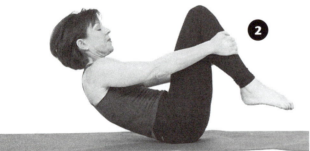

GOLF BENEFITS

• Strengthens the abdominals and pelvic floor for a stronger stance in any stroke.

stability & strength series
spine stretch forward
target: core, back

99

This classical spine series is designed to lengthen and strengthen your core muscles, especially in rotation.

STARTING POSITION: Sit with your legs extended in front of you; use a prop if necessary to insure you are in neutral spine angle. Extend your arms in front of you shoulder-width apart; keep your shoulders away from your ears throughout the movement. Imagine you are sitting at a table with your belly at the edge of the table and your hands on the tabletop. **INHALE** to begin while lengthening your spine toward the ceiling.

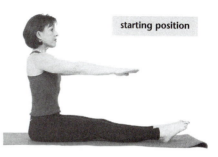

starting position

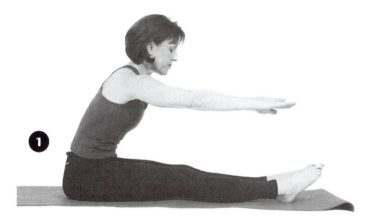

1 EXHALE and, without touching your belly to the edge, slide your hands toward the far side of the table. The trick in this movement is to keep your pelvis upright and rely on abdominal and pelvic-floor strength. Stretch yourself forward by lengthening your spine, not letting your shoulders slide up around your ears. Don't let your chin slide forward.

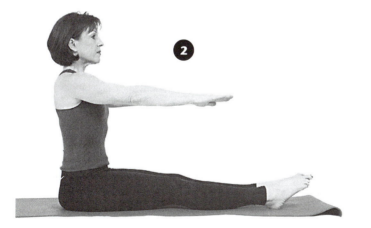

2 INHALE a sip of air then **EXHALE**, drawing in your navel to stack up the vertebrae of your spine like building blocks.

Repeat 6 times.

GOLF BENEFITS
- Stretches the muscles in the back that support the spine.
- Elongates the spine for greater rotational ability and injury prevention.

Before rotating, elongate your spine first, then activate your core muscles to keep your spine long. You'll be able to increase rotation while protecting your spine.

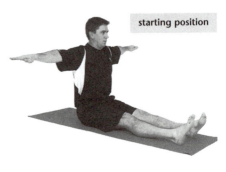

starting position

STARTING POSITION: Sit with your legs extended hip-width apart in front of you. Extend your arms out to your sides in a "T," fingertips lined up with your shoulders; keep your shoulders relaxed and your back strong throughout the movement. Imagine you are buried in sand from your pelvis to your toes. **INHALE** to begin while lengthening your spine to the ceiling.

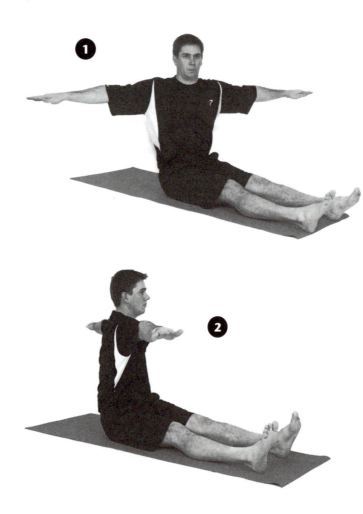

1 EXHALE while turning your upper body to the right, pulsing 2 times. Keep your weight balanced on both buttocks when you turn. Use the second pulse to squeeze the last bit of air from your lungs. Don't lean in the direction you are turning or let your fingers travel forward of your shoulder.

2 INHALE back to center, lengthening your spine again then exhaling to the left, pulsing 2 times.

Repeat the breath and movement 10 times to each side.

GOLF BENEFITS

- Builds strength in the pelvis for greater power through rotation.
- Increases flexibility in rotation for a bigger turn.

Before rotating, elongate your spine first, then activate your core muscles to keep your spine long. You'll be able to increase rotation while protecting your spine.

STARTING POSITION: Sit with your legs extended in front of you, hip-width apart. Extend your arms out to your sides in a "T," fingertips lined up with your shoulders; keep your shoulders relaxed and your hips and pelvis upright throughout the movement. **INHALE** while stretching your spine up and away from your pelvis.

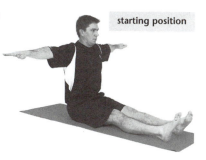

starting position

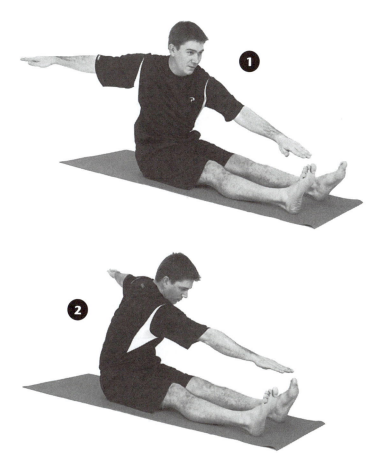

1 **EXHALE** and twist and rotate from your waistline to your right, pretending to reach your left fingertips to your right little toe. Scoop and hollow out your lower abdomen while lengthening forward.

2 **INHALE** back to center, lengthening your spine again, then **EXHALE** to repeat to the left, reaching your right fingertips toward your left little toe.

Repeat 10 times to each side.

GOLF BENEFITS
- Builds strength in the pelvis for greater power through rotation.
- Increases flexibility in rotation for a bigger turn.

stability & strength series
102
pendulum
target: core, obliques

The challenge in this exercise is keeping the opposing shoulder and hip on the floor. My scratch golfers swear by this one! If this exercise is too difficult, you can execute the movement with bent knees.

STARTING POSITION: Begin in Knees to Ceiling position, then extend your legs diagonally. Press your inner thighs, knees and ankles together and maintain neutral spine angle; imagine your legs are laced together and you have one leg instead of two. Extend your arms out to your sides; keep your shoulders and neck relaxed throughout the exercise. **INHALE** to begin.

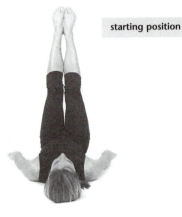

starting position

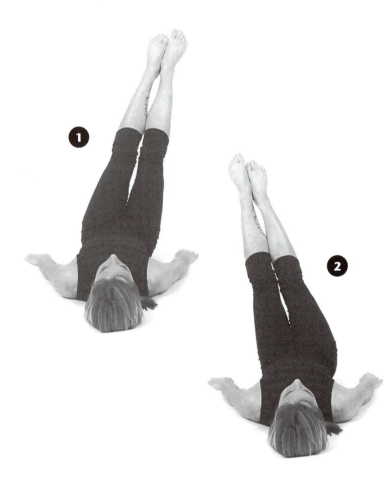

1 Keeping your shoulders and left hip on the floor, **EXHALE** and let your legs fall to the right. Don't compromise your ability to keep your opposing shoulder and hip on the floor for a larger movement of your legs.

2 **INHALE** to return to center, then **EXHALE** and let your legs fall to the left, keeping your shoulders and right hip on the floor.

Repeat right to left, counting 10 times in each direction.

GOLF BENEFITS
- Lengthens and strengthens the core.
- Stretches the back muscles.
- Enhances flexibility and power in rotation.

This is simple, but not easy, when done correctly. The challenge in this exercise is to maintain neutral spine angle while working your abdominals; do not allow the angle to change throughout the exercise. Try it while looking in a mirror, or have someone watch you to be sure you are not changing your spine angle.

STARTING POSITION: Begin in Hands and Knees position. Make sure to maintain your spine angle throughout the movement. Keep your forehead parallel to the floor and fix your gaze on a spot to avoid dropping your head forward. Keep your shoulders down and back.

starting position

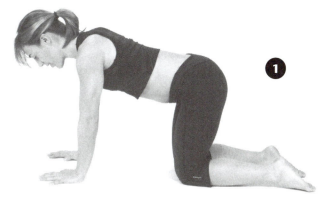

1 INHALE while completely relaxing your abdominal muscles, but don't let your spine sag toward the floor.

2 EXHALE to a slow count of **8**, drawing your abdominal muscles up toward the ceiling and compressing them against your spine. Don't round toward the ceiling when activating your abs— keep neutral spine angle.

Repeat 10 times.

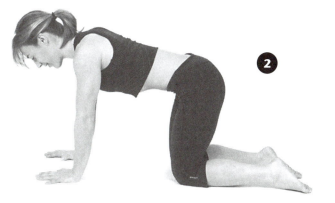

GOLF BENEFITS

- Develops muscular strength and endurance for maintaining proper spine angle.
- Increases power transfer from core to club.

ab lift with leg extension   *target: abs, shoulders, hips*

One of the best core stability exercises, this strengthens the Posterior Sling, a system of muscle and connective tissue that runs diagonally from shoulder to opposite hip, like a giant X on your back.

STARTING POSITION: Begin in Hands and Knees position. Make sure to maintain your spine angle throughout the movement. **INHALE** to begin.

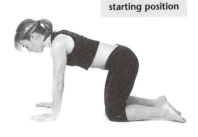

starting position

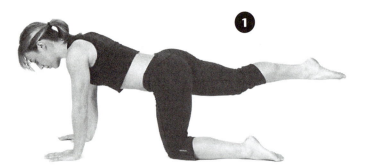

1 **EXHALE**, drawing your abdominal muscles up toward the ceiling while extending your right leg straight back to the wall behind you, lifting it to hip height.

2 **INHALE** to return to start position, then **EXHALE** and repeat with the left leg.

Repeat 10 times with each leg.

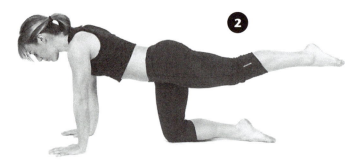

GOLF BENEFITS

• Strengthens your stance and the ability to maintain neutral spine angle in all phases of the swing.

cobra

A wonderful integrated exercise.

STARTING POSITION: Begin in Belly-Down position with both arms along your sides. Make fists with your hands and rotate your arms at your shoulders so your thumbs are pointing away from your sides, as if you were hitchhiking. Keep your head aligned. **INHALE** to begin.

starting position

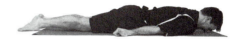

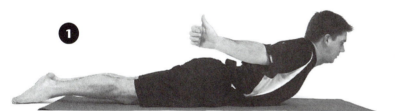

1 EXHALE while lifting your upper body, lower body and arms toward the ceiling. Try to rotate your thumbs to point to the ceiling when you lift. Hold for a full inhale. Don't compress your lower back; protect it by using your abdominal core and pelvic floor muscles.

2 EXHALE and release.

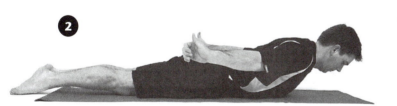

GOLF BENEFITS

• Strengthens the weaker areas of the back for a stronger and smoother swing while protecting the lower back from injury and pain.

double heel kicks
target: back, buttocks, neck

Caution: If your lower back hurts, be sure you are keeping your pelvis properly positioned on the floor and your lower abs and pelvic floor engaged. If discomfort persists, discontinue this movement until your lower abdominals are stronger.

starting position

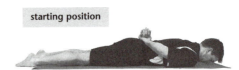

STARTING POSITION: Begin in Belly-Down position and place your forehead on the floor. Clasp your left wrist with your right hand behind your back, then bend your elbows and inch your arms up your back toward your shoulder blades. Roll your shoulders back as you extend your arms to lift and open your chest. Relax your elbows toward the floor. Keep your lower back lengthened during this movement, using your pelvic floor and abdominal lift to support the lower back.

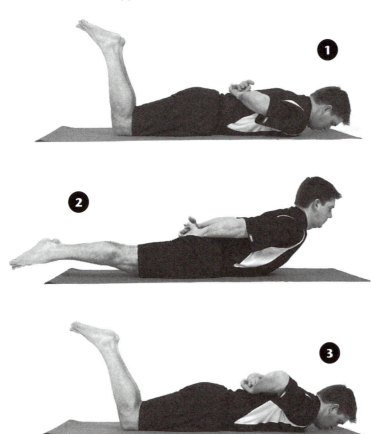

1 As you **INHALE** two short "sniffing" breaths, kick your heels toward your buttocks with 2 pulses, matching your kicks with your breath. Don't allow your hips to lift from the floor when you kick.

2 As you **EXHALE** fully, extend your legs and arms behind you and raise your chest off the floor. Imagine you are long and aerodynamic.

3 **INHALE** and bend your arms and legs back into the start position, forehead to the floor.

Repeat 10 times to each side.

GOLF BENEFITS

• Strengthens the weaker areas of the back for a stronger and smoother swing while protecting the lower back from injury and pain.

stability & strength series
mermaid
target: core, sides of waist

107

STARTING POSITION: Sit on your sitting bones with your knees bent in front of you, then drop both knees to the right. Keep your hips level and facing forward throughout the movement; use a prop under your left hip if necessary. Keep your eyes forward as if looking at the horizon to maintain neutral spine angle. Place your fingers behind your head. **INHALE** while elongating your spine.

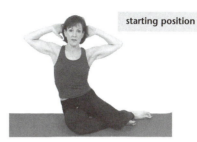

starting position

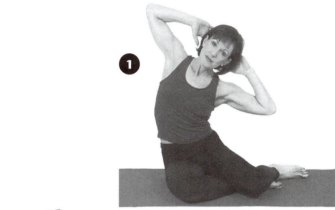

1

1 **EXHALE** and bend your torso up and over to the right. Elongate your spine, keeping the sides lifted away from your pelvis even as you are bending. Don't twist your upper body forward or backward, and don't collapse into the side you are bending toward.

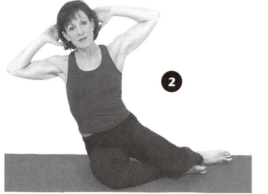

2

2 **INHALE** back to center, elongating again, then **EXHALE** and bend your torso up and over to the left.

Repeat the side-to-side movement, 10 to each side. Then fold your legs to your left and repeat.

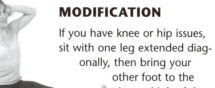

MODIFICATION

If you have knee or hip issues, sit with one leg extended diagonally, then bring your other foot to the inner thigh of the extended leg.

GOLF BENEFITS

• Greater strength and flexibility in the hips and torso make for a bigger and more powerful swing.

STARTING POSITION: Lie on your back in neutral spine angle, with knees bent and arms extended toward your toes. Extend your left leg along the floor. Maintaining neutral spine angle, extend your right leg toward the ceiling. Imagine you have a hot cup of coffee on your belly; keep your pelvis still so the coffee does not spill. **INHALE** to begin.

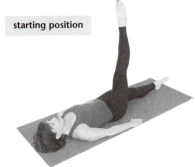

starting position

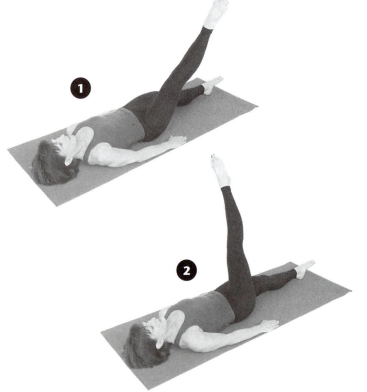

1 **EXHALE** and circle your right leg clockwise, as if you are drawing a circle on the ceiling. Imagine you are moving the bone of your upper thigh around in the hip joint, like stirring a wooden spoon around in a bowl. Move slowly through the areas where your movement is not fluid. Don't sacrifice the stability of your pelvis to make larger circles. Keep your circles small until you develop the strength to keep your pelvis still.

2 **INHALE** halfway through your circle and **EXHALE** to finish.

Repeat 8 circles and change directions. Then switch sides.

MODIFICATION

If your hips and thighs are tight, bend your knee to the ceiling. Focus on keeping your thigh relaxed.

ADVANCED

If you can circle your leg without spilling your coffee, challenge your core by making larger circles.

GOLF BENEFITS

• Increases range of motion in the hips while strengthening the core, making for a more powerful transfer of energy through the swing.

This is a great core challenge.

STARTING POSITION: Lie on your back in neutral spine angle, legs extended to the ceiling and arms out to your sides. Keep your hips and shoulders in contact with the floor throughout the exercise, and keep your inner thighs, knees and ankles pressing together. Imagine your legs are bound together and cannot come apart. Keep your arms actively engaged, drawing your shoulders down your back for core support. Keep your neck lengthened and your chin away from the ceiling.

starting position

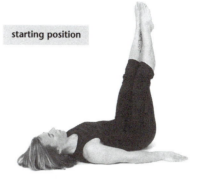

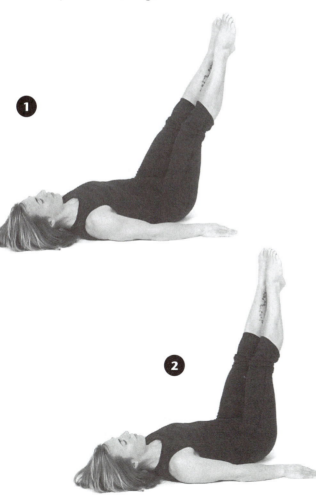

1 **INHALE** and make a circle with both legs, beginning to the right, then away from your head. Don't allow your neck and shoulders to take over the work of the pelvis.

2 **EXHALE** and continue the circle to your left and back to center. **INHALE** then change direction, moving to the left and down, then exhaling around to the right and back to center.

Count 16 circles

GOLF BENEFITS

• A great oblique abdominal strengthener that builds a stronger and more powerful turn.

STARTING POSITION: Lie on your right side, keeping your hips stacked and your upper body quiet throughout the movement. Place your top hand on the floor for support. Lengthen then lift your left leg up to approximately hip height; keep your leg extended throughout the movement. Don't allow your lower ribs to sink toward the floor. Draw your shoulders down into your back.

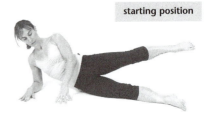

starting position

1

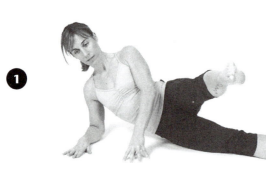

1 **INHALE** and circle your left leg forward and then toward the ceiling. Don't allow your hips to roll forward and back with the movement of your leg.

2 **EXHALE** to complete the circle to the rear and return to center.

Repeat 10 times and then reverse direction. Then switch sides.

MODIFICATION

Extend the top arm from the shoulder to point directly in front of you at shoulder height. Hold it still during the movement.

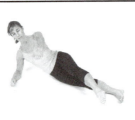

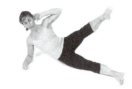

ADVANCED

Bend the top elbow and place your hand behind your head throughout the movement.

GOLF BENEFITS

• Enhances strength in the stance and fluid rotation through the hips.

stability & strength series
up and down
target: hips, legs

111

STARTING POSITION: Lie on your right side, keeping your hips stacked and your upper body quiet throughout the movement. Keep your ribcage lifting toward the ceiling. **INHALE** to begin.

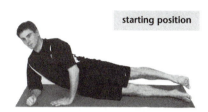

starting position

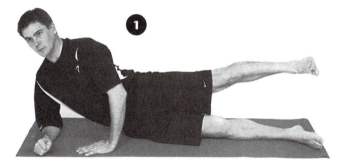

1

1 EXHALE while lengthening your left leg out of the hip joint and then up toward the ceiling; keep your thigh, knee and foot facing forward rather than toward the ceiling. Don't allow your working leg to rotate.

2 INHALE while slowly returning your leg to the start position.

Count 10 and change sides.

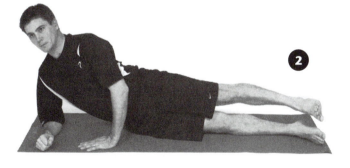

2

GOLF BENEFITS

• Prevents hip sway during weight shift because the muscle and connective tissue in the outer hip area act as a kind of retaining wall.

STARTING POSITION: Begin in a kneeling lunge with your right knee in front of your right hip, the right ankle directly under the knee. Your left knee should be directly under your left hip, with your left foot lined up behind your knee. Press the toes of your left foot into the floor. Keep your weight evenly distributed between your front and back legs throughout the movement.

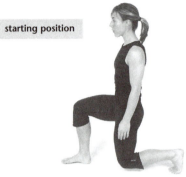

starting position

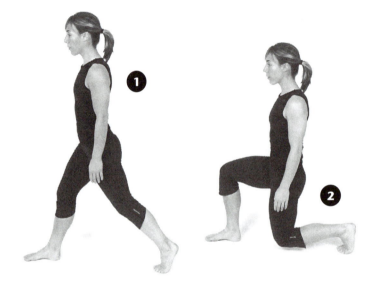

1 **INHALE** and then **EXHALE**, activating your core and buttocks muscles as you press into your feet to straighten your legs. Keep neutral spine angle (no duck butts!). Don't lean your weight forward into your front leg, and don't look down while you are in the movement. If you want to check your position, do so at the top or the bottom of the movement.

2 **INHALE** to slowly return to starting position.

Repeat 8 times on each leg.

MODIFICATION

From the starting position, place both hands on your forward knee and press up to standing as noted. Lower just a few inches toward the floor, then press up again. As your strength and balance increase, lower further toward the floor.

ADVANCED

When you reach the standing position, press off your back foot and step forward into an upright stance. Alternate legs by stepping back with the other foot.

GOLF BENEFITS

- This compound movement improves balance and is one of the best ways to strengthen your stance in any phase of the swing.
- Promotes fluid weight shift.
- Eliminates the habit of standing up in your swing.

Every aspect of the golf game involves balance. Balancing exercises require subtle precision, intense focus and relaxed, yet energized movement. Balancing exercises integrate your mind, body and emotions into a singular intention so that all of your energy is synergistically engaged for your game. This exercise trains the proper foundation for standing balance work.

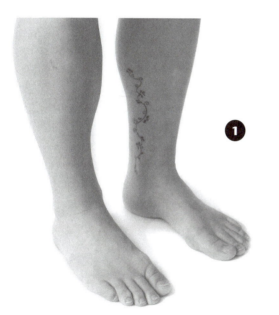

1 Breathing continuously, imagine you have old-fashioned roller skates on and balance on all four wheels. The front two wheels are on the inside and outside of the widest part of the ball of your foot; the back two wheels are on the inside and outside of your heel below your ankle.

- Feel for equal weight on both feet:
- Front to back
- Inside edge of your foot to outside edge of your foot
- Between your right and left foot.

Give your feet a solid foundation by lifting your arches slightly—imagine you have a thumbtack underneath each arch, and keep lifting away from the tack.

STARTING POSITION: Begin in Standing Balance position in front of a full-length mirror. Keep your eyes looking forward rather than at your feet. Shift your weight onto your right leg, keeping it straight but not locked. **INHALE** to begin.

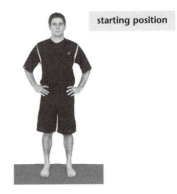

starting position

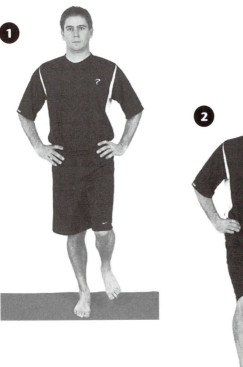

1

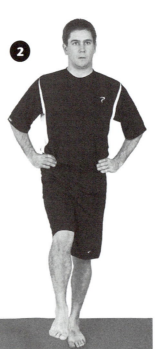

2

1 **EXHALE** while lifting your left knee. Hold for 15 seconds. Imagine your standing leg is strong and straight like a lamppost.

2 **INHALE** to replace your left leg in the starting position then shift your weight into it, keeping it straight but not locked. **EXHALE** while lifting your right knee. Hold for 15 seconds.

Continue shifting and holding, repeating 10 times on each leg. As you gain balance, increase the time until you can balance on each leg for 1 minute. Count 5 each leg.

MODIFICATION

If this is challenging, keep the toes of the bent knee close to the floor. Touch them to the floor if needed for balance.

GOLF BENEFITS

• Strengthens the entire system for balance.

Adding movement increases the challenge to the standing balance work.

STARTING POSITION: Begin in Standing Balance position.

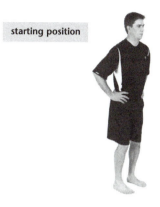

starting position

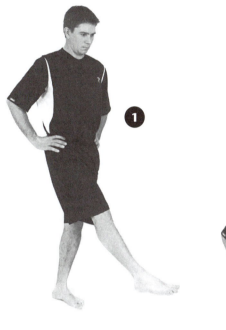

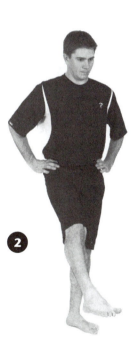

1 Shift your weight onto your left leg and extend your right leg forward at a diagonal. Relax and allow your weight to root into your standing leg. Maintain neutral spine angle throughout the movement; imagine your spine is a plumb line that is suspended from the ceiling.

2 Breathe continuously as you draw a small clockwise circle with your extended leg.

Count 10 circles and then circle counterclockwise for a count of 10. Switch sides and repeat.

MODIFICATION

If you are unable to maintain your balance and your spine angle, try making your circles smaller, focusing on balance first.

GOLF BENEFITS

• Teaches you to remain balanced on one leg while other parts of your body are moving.

standing balance series
ice skater
target: *core stability, hips*

116

This combines movement with balance for an additional challenge.

STARTING POSITION: Begin in Standing Balance position with your hands on your hips. Keep your head, chest and pelvis aligned, and keep your shoulders and hips facing straight ahead to maintain spine angle. **INHALE** to begin.

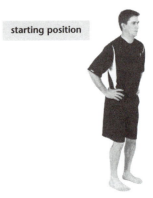

starting position

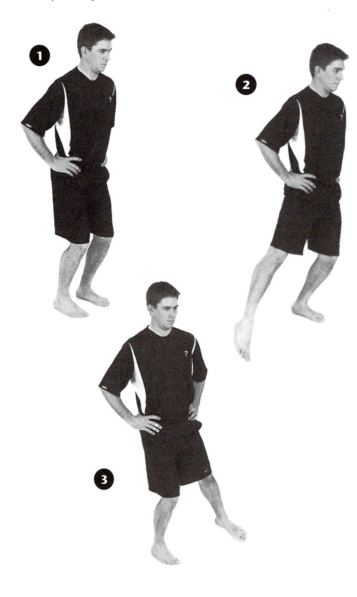

1 **EXHALE** and activate your core muscles while bending your knees and hips into a squat position. Don't look down or you'll lose your spine angle and your balance.

2 **INHALE** and shift your weight onto your left leg, then **EXHALE** and slide your right foot out to the side.

3 **INHALE** and slide your right foot back into start position, then **EXHALE** to slide your left foot out to the side. Imagine you're an ice skater, balancing on one skate as the other leg extends to push off.

Alternate shifting weight and extending legs for a total of 10.

GOLF BENEFITS

• Teaches you to maintain your spine angle and balance while shifting your weight.

single-leg twist   target: core stability, obliques

This increases the balance challenge by adding rotation.

STARTING POSITION: Stand on your left leg and raise your right knee to hip height. Raise your arms to shoulder height into a "T," keeping your hands in your peripheral vision. **INHALE** to begin.

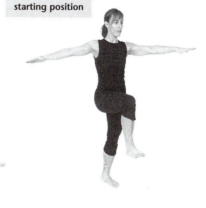

starting position

1 **EXHALE** and, while keeping your hips and legs facing forward, twist your upper body to the right. Turn your head with your upper body. Don't let your arms travel forward of your chest. Imagine your standing leg is solid like a concrete pillar and your upper body is spiraling around it.

2 **INHALE** to return to center.

3 **EXHALE** and twist to the left.

Repeat 8 times to each side, then switch sides and repeat.

GOLF BENEFITS

• Strengthens your ability to maintain balance and spine angle while rotating.

on the

green

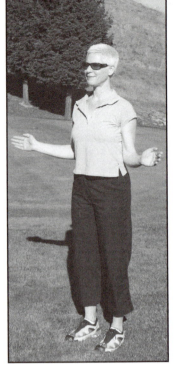

game-day plan

I run a national instructor-training program that teaches Pilates instructors how to work with golfers. I love receiving emails from instructors who are excited to relate their success stories to me. Pam had been a golf-specific Pilates instructor for about six months when she wrote. A senior golfer she had been working with for a number of months had initially signed up for ten sessions but just kept coming back for more.

Evidently, his game had improved so much that he was keeping his training a secret from his playing buddies. Even better, he said he was winning all the money, so there was no way he was letting anyone in on his secret!

This section is about optimizing your performance before, during and after your play. These tips will prepare your body and mind, increase your mental and physical stamina, and help you release

any residual tightness that might've built up from your game day.

Pre-Game Routine

Eat a good, balanced breakfast and make sure to pack some healthy snacks to take with you.

Spend about half an hour doing some breathing and active flexibility training (such as the neck stretches, shoulder and/or arm circles and knee overs) and the following Pilates

exercises to activate your core. Be sure not to fatigue your core muscles—they just need to be stimulated and awakened!

- The Hundred
- Single-leg stretch
- Cobra
- Spine Twist
- Weight Shift

Juicing the Joints

If you're like most golfers, you spend the first four holes or so warming up and getting a "feel" for your swing and for

ACTIVATE YOUR CORE

	PAGE	EXERCISE
	96	the hundred
	97	single-leg stretch
	105	cobra
	100	spine twist
	114	weight shift

pre-game routine

- increase range of motion for swing power
- decrease potential for injury
- cut strokes from your score
- find your tempo prior to play
- stimulate muscle memory to re-create your best swing.

In Play

Giving your attention to a few details can make a very big difference in your play. Here are some ways to keep your mind and body energized for the duration of your game.

Snacks

Just a small change in your blood sugar levels can alter your ability to stay focused and energized. To maintain optimal

the course. You can eliminate those additional "warm up" strokes and get a head start on your play by prepping your mind and body prior to play. The pre-swing warm-ups (pages 124–30) will prepare you body for golf movement prior to hitting at the range or at the course. They should be done no more than half an hour prior to play.

Warm-ups such as Arm Circles and Swinging Gate prepare the shoulders for the swing. The rotating movements of Washing Machine, both Helicopters and Around the World ready the torso for the full-body exertion of golf. The Windmill with Club sets up your tempo and swing.

Once you know the pre-swing routine by heart, it will take four to five minutes to complete, but it will save you four or five strokes in the end. Think of yourself like the Tin Man from *The Wizard of Oz*. He had to have his joints lubricated with oil or he became stiff and unable to move. We need the same kind of lubrication for our joints.

We have a joint-lubricating "juice" that is emitted when we move the joints through range of motion. I call it "juicing the joints." Because the exercises help you develop your sense of tempo, you'll find that you'll become very relaxed while you do them. You can use one or two of them between holes to stay relaxed and in your rhythm. By taking a few moments and juicing your joints prior to play, you can:

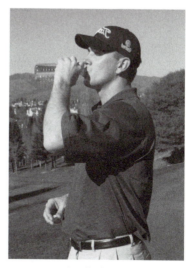

Stay hydrated!

blood sugar levels, keep some balanced snacks with you. Balance™ bars and other snack bars are designed to keep your blood sugar levels even and are a good choice for golfers.

Hydration

Staying hydrated is another way to keep your edge while playing. Studies show that many people are chronically dehydrated, and dehydration has dramatic effects on performance. Keep bottled water with you at all times and be sure to drink at least eight cups of water a day. Sports drinks are generally not the best choice for hydration due to their high sugar content, which will spike the blood sugar. Personally, I like SmartWater™, which is a puri-fied source of water that is enhanced with electrolytes.

Save your soles

You can ease the wear and tear on your feet, ankles, legs, hips and back with a good insole. Sports insoles are widely avail-able at running stores and

outdoor sports stores. A good insole can decrease stress to your lower body and back up to 40 percent.

Use your legs

Use good body mechanics when you retrieve your ball or pick up your bag. Protect your lower back by engaging your abdominal core, and use your legs, rather than your lower back, to bend.

Enjoy the sun safely

Use sunblock, a hat and sports glasses that protect your eyes. There are some great outdoor clothing lines that make sun-protective clothing. See the Resource list.

Post-Game

I don't expect you to walk off the course and immediately start a post-game cool-down; after all, you'll be collecting your earnings and gloating over your new game! Any time before you go to bed is fine.

Spend about 20 minutes on a combination of roller release work and flexibility exercises

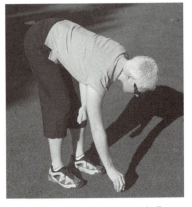

Incorrect way to pick up a ball

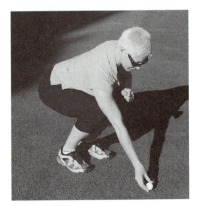

Correct way to pick up a ball

(pages 71–87). You can tailor your post-game program to your needs, focusing on where you tend to tighten. The static flexibility exercises are relaxing, so doing them just before you go to bed is a good way to pre-pare for a good night's sleep.

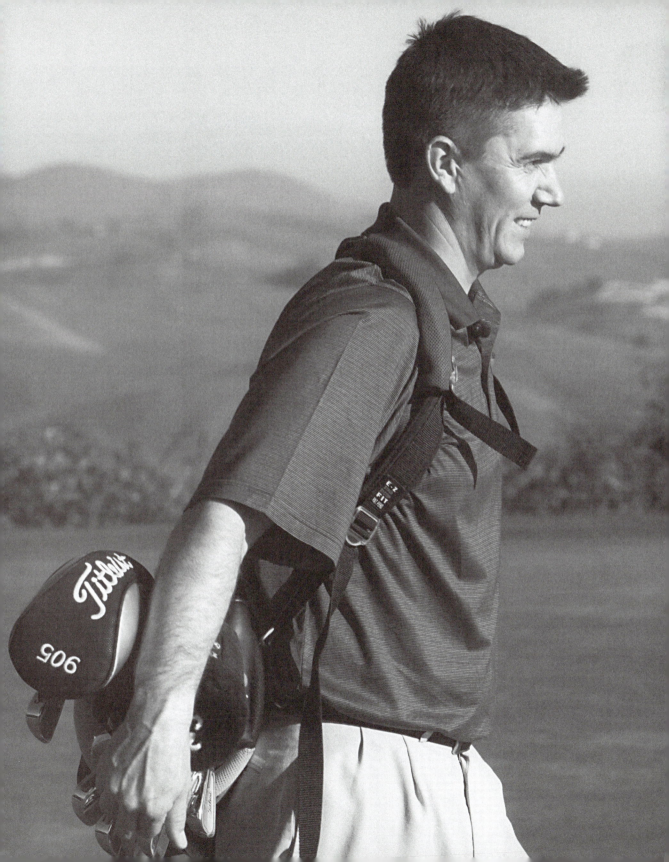

arm circles

If you have a shoulder issue or any pain, bend your elbow and start with small circles. If pain persists, have your shoulder checked out by a professional.

STARTING POSITION: Begin in address stance with neutral spine angle and your arms at your sides. Breathe continuously and keep your torso still throughout the exercise.

starting position

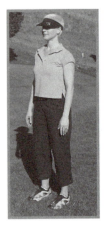

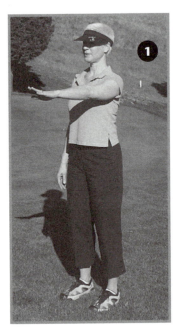

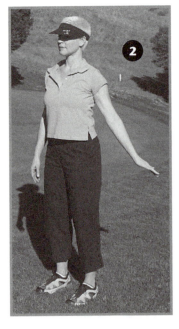

1 Draw a continuous, fluid circle with your left arm by extending it forward, and then up toward the sky.

2 Continue circling your arm up and back behind you in a large arc. Don't twist your torso in order to make larger circles. Repeat 6 times.

Then circle the arm 6 times in the opposite direction before switching arms.

GOLF BENEFITS
- Prepares the rotator cuff muscles for the golf swing.
- Increases shoulder turn.

STARTING POSITION: Stand in address stance with neutral spine angle. Bend your arms so that your forearms are parallel to the ground. Imagine your elbows are pinned to your sides by a hinge, like a gate attached to a post. Keep them close to your body during the movement.

starting position

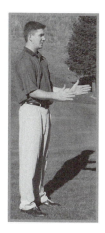

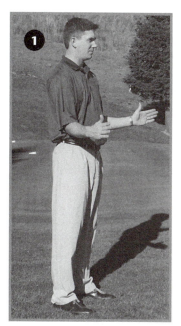

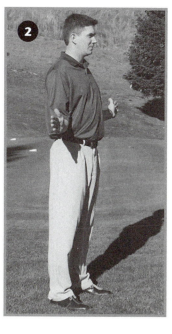

1 Breathing continuously, smoothly open your arms out to the sides.

2 Once you've reached the limit of your range of motion, return to center and repeat 10 times.

GOLF BENEFITS

- Increases shoulder and torso flexibility for a bigger, better swing.
- Prepares your takeaway arm to rotate for proper position in the backswing.
- Helps keep you on your swing plane.
- Keeps the non-target-side elbow in place during the backswing and follow-through.

washing machine

STARTING POSITION: Stand in address stance with neutral spine angle. Make fists and bend your arms so that your forearms are parallel to the ground. Keep your elbows glued to your sides throughout the exercise.

starting position

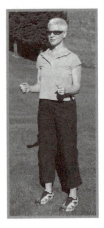

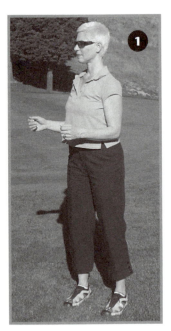

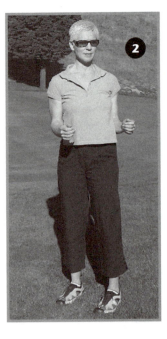

1 Breathing continuously and keeping your pelvis still, rotate your arms and torso to the right. Imagine that your torso is the agitator in a washing machine. Allow your head and neck to move with your torso.

2 Return to center to rotate to the left.

Repeat 10 times to each side.

GOLF BENEFITS

- Increases rotation for a fuller swing.
- Protects the lower back from injury.

STARTING POSITION: Stand in address stance with neutral spine angle. Lift your arms out to your sides into a "T," keeping your fingers aligned with your collarbones. Breathe continuously throughout the movement.

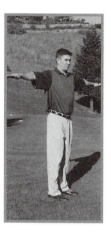

starting position

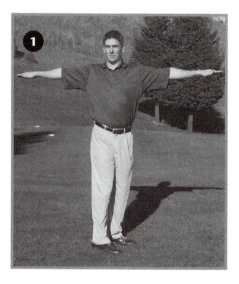

1 Keeping your lower body stable and your fingers in line with your collarbones, rotate your upper body to the right.

2 Smoothly rotate back to center and continue to the left.

Do 10 to each side.

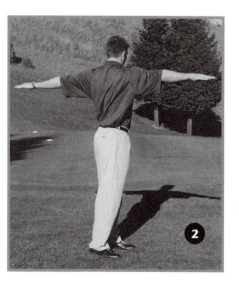

GOLF BENEFITS

• Increases trunk rotation for a fuller, more fluid swing.

helicopters with lunge

STARTING POSITION: Begin in a lunge position with your front knee directly over your front ankle. Bring your arms out to your sides in a "T," lining up your fingers with your collarbones. Make sure your heel and toes are lined up facing straight ahead. Breathe continuously throughout the movement.

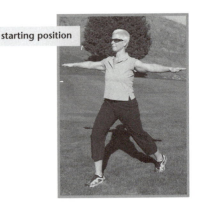

starting position

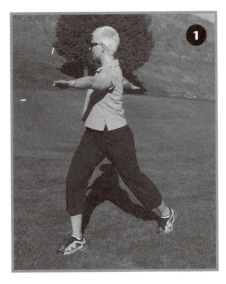

1 Keeping the hips still and your pelvis facing forward throughout the exercise, rotate your arms and twist through your torso to the right. Don't lean forward over your front leg or let your front knee travel beyond your front toes. Keep your fingers in line with your collarbones.

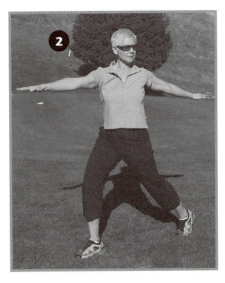

2 Smoothly rotate and twist through the center to the left.

Do 10 to each side and then switch legs so the other foot is in front.

GOLF BENEFITS

• Increases range of motion through the torso for enhanced hip and shoulder turn. Challenges balance for enhanced weight shift.

STARTING POSITION: Stand in address stance with neutral spine angle and raise your hands over your head. Clasp one wrist in the opposite hand. Breathe continuously throughout the movement.

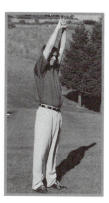

starting position

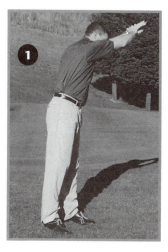

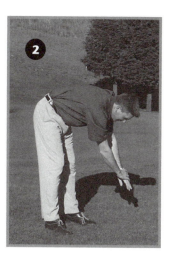

1 Start drawing a large circle with your arms by bending to the left as far as you can go.

2 Continue the circle, bending forward as you come over your feet. Allow your knees to bend if necessary and release your head to the floor.

3 Continue crossing your body to come up the other side.

Repeat 6 times then switch directions.

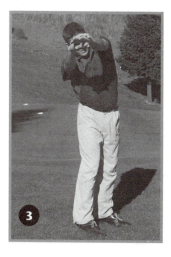

GOLF BENEFITS

- Increases range of motion through the hips, shoulders and torso for maximum movement and power in the swing.

windmill with club

I learned this one from Dr. Joseph Parent, the Zen Golf™ Coach. This exercise really puts it all together prior to play. Left-handed golfers: Make the necessary changes to the hands and the position of the club.

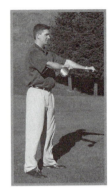

STARTING POSITION: Begin in address stance in neutral spine angle. Hold your driver parallel to the ground with the club head pointing to your right. Place your left hand, palm down, on the grip. Place your right hand, palm up, on the shaft as close to the club-head end as comfortable. Breathe continuously.

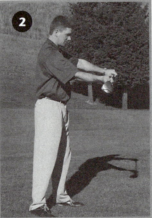

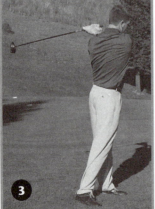

1 Rotate your torso to the left and then the right, as in the Washing Machine exercise—the club will travel in a circular motion around you.

2 Each time you rotate to the left, move your right palm up the shaft toward your left hand.

3 Count 10 rotations, bringing your palms together. The placement of your hands will eventually end up resembling your golf grip.

Continue moving the club around yourself, rolling the arms to open the club to the right and close the club when it moves to your left. Count another 10 rotations.

GOLF BENEFITS
• Sets your tempo and your swing prior to stepping up to the tee.

chest stretch

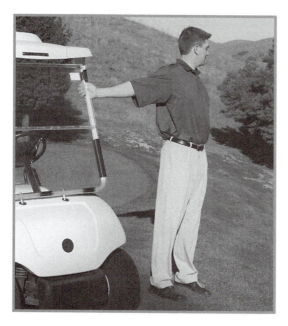

Grasp the riser with one hand at about shoulder height. Stand at arm's length away from the riser. Breathe while gently turning your body away from the riser to stretch the front shoulder and chest muscles. Relax the neck and upper body. Keep your spine aligned

Breathing continuously, hold the stretch for 60 seconds.

lower back stretch

Facing your golf cart, grasp the riser with both hands, placing them below the level of your shoulders. Draw your navel to your spine, bend your knees and bend forward from your hips. Round your lower spine. Breathing continuously, hold the stretch for 60 seconds.

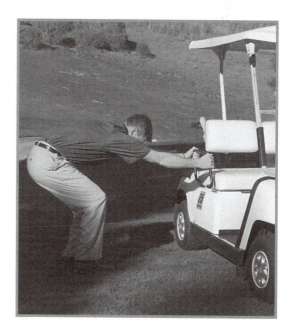

calf stretch

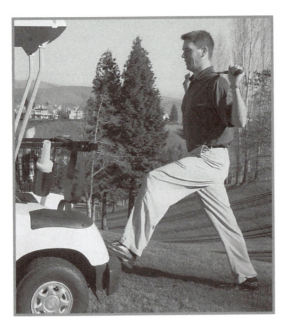

Place one foot on the cart floor or the bumper, aligning your hip, knee and toe. Lengthen and align the back leg into a lunge position, keeping your heel down. Keep your spine angle in neutral and your hips facing forward. Exhale and draw your navel to your spine, lengthening your lower back. Breathing continuously, hold the stretch for 60 seconds. Repeat on the other side.

hamstring stretch

Facing your golf cart, place one hand on the cart for support as you bend forward. Flex the toes of one foot back toward the knee; grasp the toes with the same side hand if possible. Find a comfortable stretch for the hamstring muscle in the back of the thigh. Breathing continuously, hold the stretch for 60 seconds. Repeat on the other side.

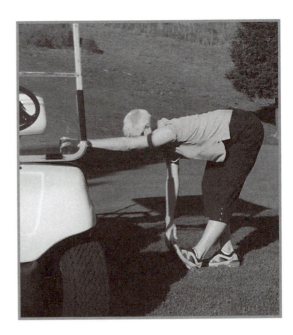

side-bending stretch

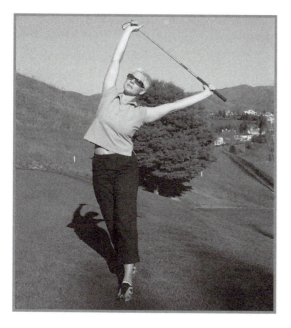

Stand with your left foot forward and your right foot slightly behind you. Hold a golf club with both hands and stretch your arms overhead. Keeping your shoulders away from your ears, lean to the left. Lift your ribcage away from your pelvis, making the sides of your torso longer. Breathing continuously, hold the stretch for 60 seconds. Switch legs and lean to the other side.

shoulder rotation stretch

Stand in neutral spine angle and face away from the cart. Reach back and behind the shoulder to hold on to the riser. Find a gentle stretch, adjusting your distance from the cart accordingly. Breathing continuously, hold the stretch for 60 seconds. Repeat on the other side.

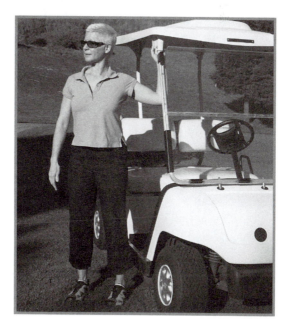

figure-four hip stretch

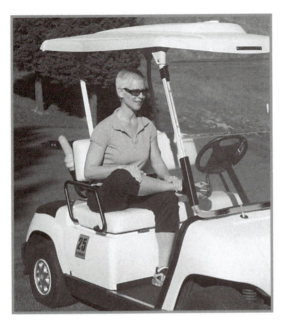

Sit tall in the golf cart and cross one ankle over the opposite thigh, just above the knee. Draw your navel to your spine and bend forward at your hips until you find a gentle stretch in your hip joint. Breathing continuously, hold the stretch for 60 seconds. Repeat on the other side.

rotation stretch

Sit tall in your golf cart and draw your navel to your spine. Inhale as you rotate your spine to the right, beginning at your lower back, working up the spine to rotate your chest, shoulders and finally neck and head. Place your left hand on the outside of your right knee to increase the stretch. Breathing continuously, hold the stretch for 60 seconds. Exhale to return to center, then repeat on the other side.

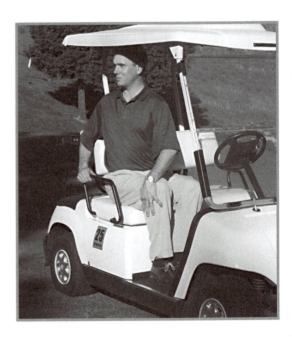

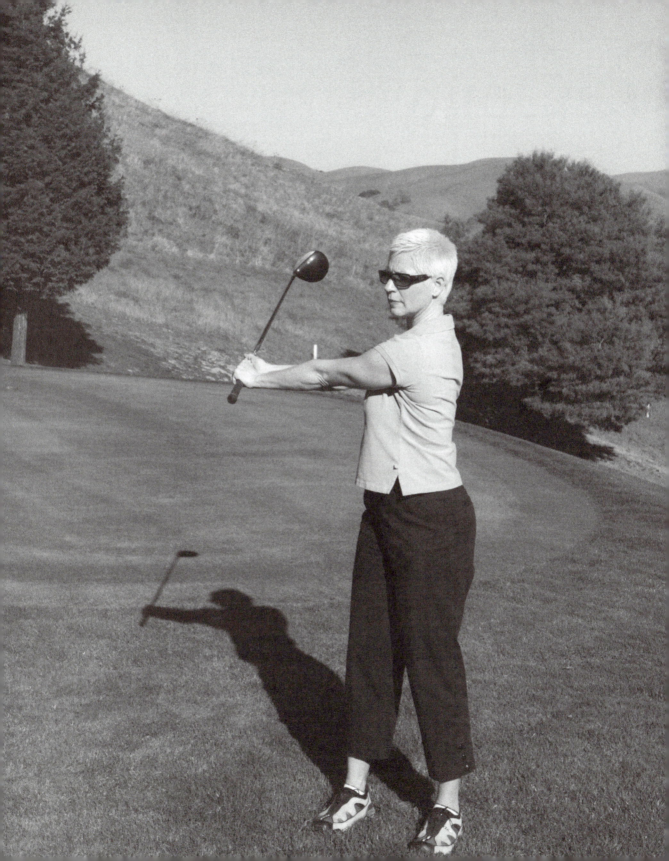

resources

Following is a list of certified Pilates for Golf Coach™ instructors. They have advanced, golf-specific training and can tailor golf-specific exercise programs designed to meet your unique movement needs.

Within the U.S.

Arizona

Barb Stephens
Mesa, AZ
e-mail: barb.stephens@asu.edu

Michelle Marking
Scottsdale, AZ
e-mail: michellemarking@earth
   link.net

California

Kris Landry (licensed)
Antioch, CA 94531
925-754-8658
e-mail: info@thepilatesolution.
   com

Lisa Sloat
Calabasas, CA
BetterBody Pilates
818-224-4734
e-mail: lisasloat@hotmail.com

Maricar Pratt
Calabasas, CA: 818-224-4734
Oak Park, CA: 818-707-3723
e-mail: mpratt@betterbody
   pilates.com

Claudia Moose
Lafayette, CA
925-299-9642
e-mail: claudia@absolute
   center.net

Katie Santos
Lafayette, CA
925-299-9642
e-mail: katie@absolute
   center.net

Peg Wallace
San Francisco, CA
e-mail: peg@elevationpilates.
   com

Jeanette Newman
Sonoma, CA
707-971-9700
e-mail: jeanette@emris.com

Aggie Winstron
Westlake Village, CA
e-mail: pawins@adelphia.net

Laurie Walker
Westlake Village, CA
ProActive Pilates
805-557-1524

Connecticut

Brian Magna
Avon, CT
e-mail: magnagolfmedicine@
   sbcglobal.net

Hawaii

Jennifer Lancaster (licensed)
Hawaii
808-756-1846
e-mail: jllart@erols.com

Kentucky

Patti Joyce
Louisville, KY
e-mail: healthymind@bell
   south.net

Massachusetts

Renee Hirl
Newton, MA
617-773-8011
e-mail: reneehirl@rcn.com

Michigan

Kelly Hale
Birmingham, MI
e-mail: funfit@ameritech.net

Barbara Hayes
Birmingham, MI
284-644-0284
e-mail: hayes4mail@aol.com

Susan Pontes
Bloomfield Hills, MI
248-642-6207

Jim Hayward
Grosse Pointe, MI
586-228-5057
e-mail: jimhayward@eaton.com

Lynn Scharret
Southfield, MI
810-625-0895

Nevada
Kimm Miller
Las Vegas, NV
e-mail: kimmfitness@aol.com

Crystal O'Shea
Las Vegas, NV
e-mail: crystal-oshea@cox.net

Kimberly Parrish
Las Vegas, NV
e-mail: pilatesgarden@earth
link.net

Suzanne Ryder
Las Vegas, NV
e-mail: purepilates@excite.com

Manodnya Vakil PT
Las Vegas, NV
e-mail: joyenv@earthlink.net

New Jersey
Barbara Hoon
Florham Park, NJ
e-mail: blini456@aol.com

New York
Anna Moy
New York, NY
e-mail: pages1212@yahoo.com

Lisa Serradilla
New York, NY
e-mail: lisa@pilatium.com

North Carolina
Leanne Case
Greensboro, NC
e-mail: lscase@uncg.edu

Ohio
Tami Singer
Cincinnati, OH
e-mail: tsing24@aol.com

Jay Apking
The Pilates Loft
Cincinnati, OH
513-351-7587
e-mail: japking@aol.com

Judi Cettel
Cincinnati, OH
e-mail: jcettel@cinci.rr.com

Diane Waring
Cincinnati, OH
e-mail: dianewaring@hillen
brand.com

Marcia Polas
Columbus, OH
e-mail: polaspilates@yahoo.com

Amy Conrad
Dayton, OH
e-mail: amyconrad@earth
link.net

Kathy Anderson
Dayton, OH
e-mail: kathyanderson@phil
herman.com

Scott Meyers and Karina
Richter
Lakewood, OH
e-mail: scottmeyers1@hot
mail.com

Tracy Ginnetti
Mainville, OH
e-mail: tginetti@cinci.rr.com

Oklahoma
Roxie Maynard
Edmond, OK
e-mail: roxamay@cox.net

Laura Foster
Tulsa, OK
e-mail: ljfoster@yahoo.com

Pennsylvania
Arlene Warunek
Gym La Femme
Pittston, PA
e-mail: awpilates@aol.com

Texas

Tracy Brewer
Arlington, TX
e-mail: tracyannbrewer@
   yahoo.com

Pam Blangy
Houston, TX
e-mail: plangy@sbcglobal.net

Patricia Schrum
Katy, TX
e-mail: pschrum@houston.
   rr.com

Rudy Peters
Richardson, TX
e-mail: rjpeters@yahoo.com

Virginia

Cherie Mooboer
Fairfax, VA
e-mail: phitnessfun@aol.com

Suzanne Miller
Haymarket, VA
e-mail: suzanne.miller@bae
   systems.com

Outside the U.S.
Canada

Phyllis Balshine
Ontario, Canada
e-mail: core.elements@
   gmail.com

England

Jean Monger
Pullborough, West Sussex
e-mail: jean4pilates@aol.com

Korea

Mark Dong Ham Kim
Seoul, Korea
e-mail: dokim77@yahoo.com

index